MRCPsych OSCEs *for* Part 1

Senior Lecturer
Imperial College
London

John Lowe
Consultant Adult Psychiatrist
St Charles Hospital
Imperial College
London

Jan Wise
Consultant Adult Psy
Park Royal Centre for
Central Middle

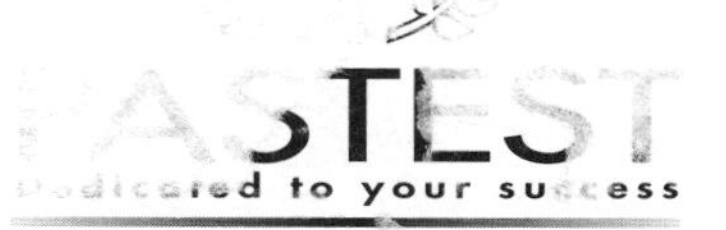

Egerton Court
Parkgate Estate
Knutsford
Cheshire, WA16 8DX

Telephone: 01565 752000

First edition 2004

ISBN: 1 904627 04 8

A catalogue record for this book is available from the British Library.

Cover design by Old Tin Dog Design Company
Typeset by Saxon Graphics Ltd, Derby
Printed by Page Bros. (Norwich Ltd)

Contents

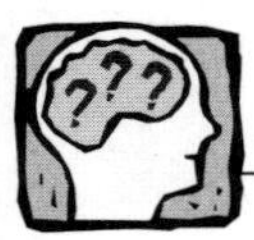

Introduction

The MRCPsych examination is now taken by more candidates than ever before. Almost 2,000 people attempt the examination every year and of these, less than half are successful.

The OSCE was introduced relatively recently in an attempt to improve the reliability of the clinical component of the examination in the face of the ever-growing numbers of candidates. It represents a significant hurdle. A quarter of those attempting the OSCE are unsuccessful and are obliged to pass the written part of the examination for a second time before being allowed to attempt the OSCE again.

Preparing for the OSCE represents a unique challenge. The most effective OSCE revision takes place in small groups and involves talking through or practising OSCE stations. There is a wide range of potential OSCEs and, although it is impossible to practise them all, there are common themes and even 'set pieces' which recur time and again.

This book covers this important area comprehensively from many different angles. Unlike other OSCE books, this book provides "instructions for actor", so that candidates can practise OSCEs with each other, by one person taking on the role of actor. The OSCEs are well constructed, give detailed background information and are well suited to practise within groups. Reading this book and practising the OSCEs will lead to a greater understanding of the variety of topics which may be covered and the possible formats of different OSCE stations. Thinking through, practising and discussing the OSCEs before the examination will improve your clarity of thought and confidence, helping you to manage your anxiety on the day of the real examination.

Using this book carefully will help you develop the required skills. You will be much better equipped to pass the OSCE and far less likely to face the unenviable task of sitting the written paper again.

Dr Nicholas Taylor MRCPsych
Author of *The A-Z for the MRCPsych*

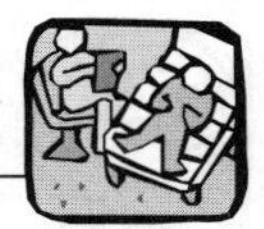

OSCE 1

Instructions for candidate

Interview this patient and look for evidence of alcohol dependence.

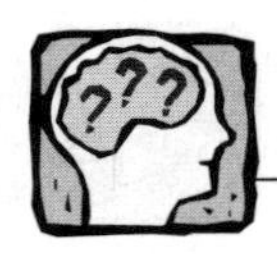

Instructions for actor

You have been referred to a psychiatrist against your will. Your wife has threatened to leave you unless you address your alcohol problems. She is fed up with your behaviour at home, as you neglect both her and your children. Although you admit that you like a drink, you do not feel that alcohol is a major problem for you.

Over the years you have developed a consistent pattern of drinking. You used to drink smaller amounts, but at work you started having drinks at lunchtime to cope with the demands of your job. You returned to work intoxicated several times and were dismissed.

Since you lost your job you have been drinking three pints of lager at lunchtime and a further five to eight pints in the evening. By midday you have a strong urge to have a drink. If you do not start drinking then, you begin to shake. Once you have that first drink your shakes diminish. You have not had a day off drinking for at least a year. On that occasion you had severe abdominal pains and brought up coffee-ground-like vomit. Once you had recovered from that episode, you rapidly started drinking heavily again.

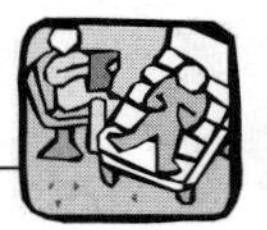

Construct

The candidate should be able to take an accurate alcohol history. The patient is reluctant to be seen, so the candidate will need to demonstrate an empathetic response. They should be able to establish the presence of alcohol dependence.

Examiner's marking sheet

	Excellent	Good	Satisfactory	Fail	Poor
Communication skills					
Taking an accurate alcohol history					
Establishing that alcohol is problematic for the patient					
Identifying the presence of alcohol dependence					
Overall mark					

Communication skills

OSCEs which have substance misuse as a theme may often contain instructions for the simulated patient to appear reluctant to be seen, or even antagonistic. Therefore you should look out for this, as you will score marks if you can demonstrate that you have elicited the patient's negative attitude.

Once you have identified the reluctance of the patient, emphasise your attempts to establish an empathetic approach.

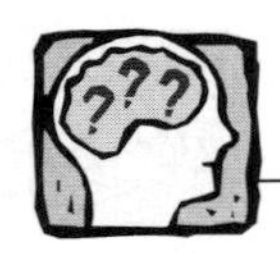

Taking an accurate alcohol history

When taking an alcohol history, you need to demonstrate to the examiner that you are aware of how units of alcohol are measured. One unit of alcohol is contained in approximately half a pint of beer, one glass of wine or one measure of spirits.

This patient drinks 8–11 pints of beer daily. This is equivalent to 16–22 units of alcohol per day or 112–154 units per week. To score maximum points in this section, calculate the units aloud for the benefit of the examiner. You could then follow this up with a health education statement. For example:

> 'From what you have told me it appears you are drinking between 100 and 150 units of alcohol per week. Are you aware that the safe recommended limits for drinking alcohol for men are a maximum of 21 units, or ten and a half pints of beer per week?'

Establishing that alcohol is problematic for the patient

This requires you to ask appropriate screening questions such as those of the CAGE questionnaire.

CAGE is an acronym for the following four questions.

1 Have you ever felt as though you needed to **c**ut down on your alcohol intake?

2 Have you ever become **a**ngry when others have criticised your drinking?

3 Have you ever felt **g**uilty about your alcohol consumption?

4 Have you ever used alcohol as an **e**ye opener (or to relieve withdrawal symptoms)?

If you receive positive responses to any of the CAGE questions, or you elicit other evidence of possible problematic drinking, you will need to examine the patient for evidence of alcohol dependence.

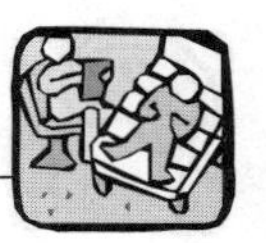

Identifying the presence of alcohol dependence

There are seven key features of alcohol dependence as originally described by Edwards and Gross. These have been incorporated into ICD-10. To establish the presence of alcohol dependence, ask about each of the following areas.

Stereotyped pattern of drinking

Whereas a social drinker may drink wine with a meal, beer in a pub, champagne on special occasions, etc, a dependent drinker tends to drink the same product in similar amounts on a daily basis. This patient's description of daily pints of beer would fit into this category.

Prominence of drink-seeking behaviour

In a dependent drinker, alcohol consumption takes priority over other activities of daily living. This situation persists even when the patient has experienced adverse outcomes of drinking.

Compulsion to drink

The dependent patient has cravings for alcohol. Once they have had one drink, they then find it very hard to stop drinking.

Withdrawal symptoms

These include tremors and nausea. More severe withdrawal symptoms include convulsions and delirium tremens.

Relief drinking

The dependent patient drinks alcohol in order to relieve or avoid the onset of withdrawal symptoms.

Development of tolerance

The dependent patient needs to consume increasing amounts of alcohol in order to obtain the same physical/psychological effects.

Reinstatement after abstinence

After a period of either voluntary or enforced abstinence, if the patient starts drinking again they rapidly return to the same pattern of consumption.

Further reading

Edwards, G. and Gross, M. 1976. Alcohol dependence: provisional description of a clinical syndrome. *British Medical Journal,* 1, 1058.

Mayfield, D., McLeod, G. and Hall, P. 1974. The CAGE questionnaire: validation of a new alcoholism screening instrument. *American Journal of Psychiatry,* 131, 1121–1123.

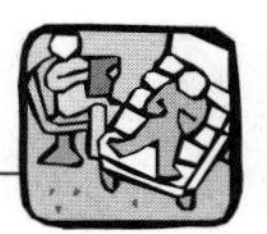

OSCE 2

Instructions for candidate

Assess the link between cannabis and this outpatient's mental illness. Provide information on the harmful effects of cannabis, and answer questions on the link between cannabis and psychosis.

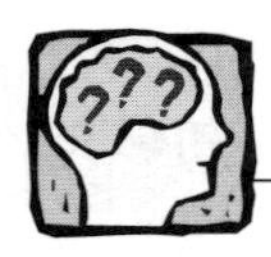

Instructions for actor

You have recently recovered from an episode of mental illness. You were under increasing amounts of stress at home and at work. You eventually became very unwell and needed to be admitted to hospital for several weeks. You now feel better and have come for a review at the outpatient clinic.

When you were ill you found that you were becoming increasingly distressed. You felt that your friends were talking about you behind your back and were deliberately trying to antagonise you. You thought that strangers were looking at you in a sinister manner when you walked past them in the street. You started to hear voices calling out unpleasant remarks about your appearance, but you could not see where the voices were coming from.

As your mental health deteriorated, in an attempt to calm yourself you started to smoke increasing amounts of cannabis. You believe that cannabis improved your mental state, as when you were intoxicated you felt relaxed.

You have continued to smoke cannabis since your discharge. When the doctor questions you about this in your appointment today, you become angry. You tell him that cannabis has been downgraded from a class B to a class C substance by the Government as it is harmless. You ask the doctor what relevance cannabis consumption has to your episode of mental illness.

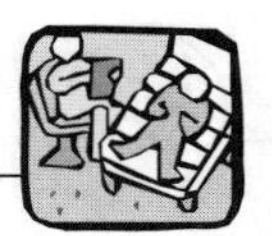

Construct

This OSCE assesses the candidate's ability to help a patient to understand the link between his cannabis misuse and his mental illness. The patient lacks insight into this issue and may exhibit anger when the link is suggested. The candidate should be able demonstrate an empathetic response to the patient.

Examiner's marking sheet

	Excellent	Good	Satisfactory	Fail	Poor
Communication skills					
Eliciting history of cannabis consumption					
Assessment of the patient's degree of insight with regard to cannabis and mental illness					
Explanation of the link between cannabis and psychosis in a manner that the patient understands					
Overall mark					

Communication skills

This OSCE tests the candidate's ability to assess insight. Once the candidate has identified the adverse prognostic factor of cannabis consumption, this link has to be made carefully, as the patient enjoys using cannabis.

In this OSCE the actor will have been briefed to become angry if the candidate says that his use of cannabis will affect his prognosis. The

OSCE therefore assesses whether the candidate can appropriately handle the patient's anger when he is challenged about his use of cannabis.

Eliciting history of cannabis consumption

The key to this part of the OSCE is to elicit the link between cannabis consumption and the patient's mental illness.

You should have some idea of how cannabis is consumed (it is usually smoked, but can be ingested). You should also have an idea of the commonly used amounts of cannabis (eg it is often bought in multiples of an eighth of an ounce). Different varieties of cannabis also differ markedly in potency. Ask about the number of joints smoked per day or the weight of cannabis consumed. Also ask whether cannabis is smoked alone or as a member of a group (in the latter case this will dilute the total quantity consumed).

The candidate should be able to elicit the fact that the patient increased his consumption of cannabis as he became unwell, as he was using the drug as a form of self-medication.

Assessment of the patient's degree of insight with regard to cannabis and mental illness

Having established that cannabis consumption increased as the patient became unwell, the candidate will need to elicit whether the patient has any awareness of the detrimental effect of cannabis on mental state.

The actor has been briefed to say that cannabis is not harmful, and that even the Government thinks so as it has downgraded the drug from a class B to a class C substance. The candidate should therefore explain that downgrading from class B to class C is a legal classification and has implications for the police and courts, but it does not mean that cannabis is not harmful to vulnerable individuals. Using the example of legal but harmful drugs such as alcohol or nicotine may help to make this point.

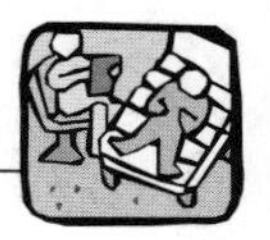

Explanation of the link between cannabis and psychosis in a manner that the patient understands

The actor has been briefed to say that taking cannabis helps him to relax. You should acknowledge to the patient that cannabis has this immediate relaxing effect on him while he is intoxicated. By doing this you will improve rapport. You should next point out that as a result of the acute intoxicating effect of cannabis, some individuals mistakenly believe that taking this drug is beneficial when they are feeling mentally unwell.

However, you then need to mention that during or after intoxication, susceptible individuals can experience heightened perceptions or psychotic phenomena, which lead to distress. This in turn leads to further cannabis consumption in an attempt to self-medicate. By entering this vicious circle, some individuals can prolong their episodes of illness. Of course this will need to be explained without using psychiatric jargon.

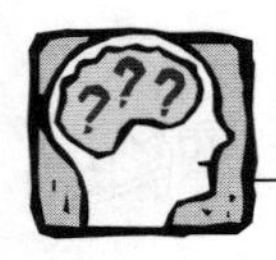

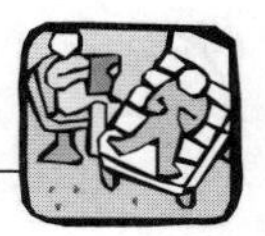

OSCE 3

Instructions for candidate

This man has presented asking for methadone. He states that he is addicted to heroin and has not had any for 24 hours. Establish that he is opiate dependent and then examine him for evidence of opiate withdrawal. Tell the examiner what you are doing.

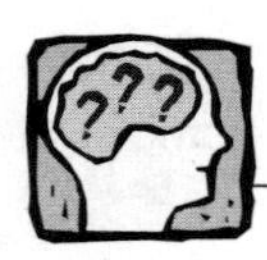

Instructions for actor

You are a heroin user in your mid-thirties. You used to smoke the drug, but have been injecting for the last two years. You try to use clean equipment, but have occasionally shared needles with other users.

You tried heroin socially at first, but you now use much more of the drug than previously. Much of your day is spent obtaining supplies and then being intoxicated. You have resorted to stealing to pay for supplies.

You spend £50 a day on the drug, which you inject, usually on two separate occasions. The effect is to make you feel relaxed, although you now need more heroin than previously in order to achieve this effect.

If you do not inject, you develop unpleasant withdrawal symptoms. These include agitation and cravings for the drug. Physically you feel unwell with a rapid heart rate, sweating, yawning, abdominal cramps and diarrhoea. Taking heroin relieves these symptoms.

You have not had any heroin for 24 hours as your dealer has been arrested. You are starting to experience the above withdrawal symptoms and are becoming agitated. You want some methadone to relieve these symptoms.

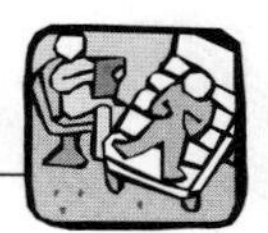

Construct

This OSCE assesses the candidate's ability to assess a distressed patient who is withdrawing from opiates. The candidate should be able to take an accurate history of opiate consumption and confirm the presence of opiate dependence, as well as assessing the patient for symptoms and signs of opiate withdrawal.

Examiner's marking sheet

	Excellent	Good	Satisfactory	Fail	Poor
Communication skills					
Eliciting history of consumption					
Assessment of opiate dependence					
Assessment of symptoms of opiate withdrawal					
Examination for evidence of opiate withdrawal					
Overall mark					

Communication skills

In this OSCE, the patient is beginning to experience withdrawal symptoms from heroin and is starting to become agitated. You should acknowledge that the patient is feeling unwell and reassure him that you will try to help to relieve his symptoms once you have completed your assessment.

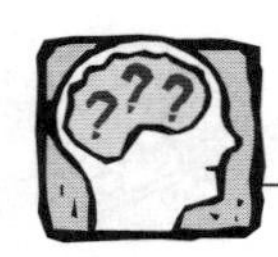

Eliciting history of consumption

As with OSCE 2, it is important to be aware of how an illicit drug such as heroin is consumed (smoked or injected), as well as the quantities in which heroin is commonly taken (bag, weight, money spent).

In this OSCE the patient injects heroin. You should therefore ask whether he has ever shared needles with other heroin users, as this of course carries the risk of bloodborne infections, in particular hepatitis B and C and HIV.

Assessment of opiate dependence

The criteria for establishing dependence are described in the answer to OSCE 1.

For opiate use in particular, prominent symptoms will include cravings, severe withdrawal symptoms and primacy of drug taking, including disregard of social and physical consequences of drug use.

Assessment of symptoms of opiate withdrawal

The candidate will need to know the common symptoms of withdrawal from opiates. They should therefore ask about the following:

- the presence of cravings
- the presence of gastrointestinal symptoms, including nausea, vomiting, cramps and diarrhoea
- the presence of any muscle or joint pains.

Examination for evidence of opiate withdrawal

An actor cannot of course simulate physical signs. However, you should examine them for the presence of the signs below. The only way in which you can demonstrate to the examiner that you know what you are looking for is by stating aloud what you are trying to elicit – for example, 'May I check your pulse to assess whether you have a fast heartbeat?'.

Signs of opiate withdrawal include the following:

- general observations – yawning, lacrimation, rhinorrhoea, sweating, agitation

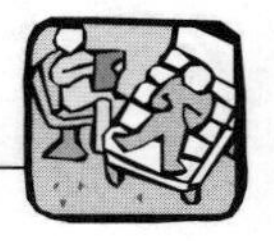

- increased body temperature, dehydration, piloerection
- cardiovascular signs – increased heart rate, increased or decreased blood pressure
- respiratory signs – increased respiratory rate
- neurological signs – dilated pupils, tremor.

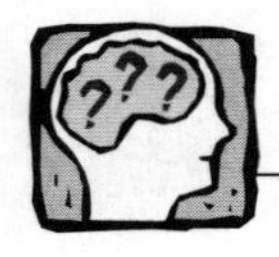

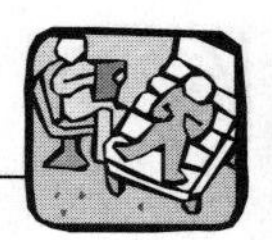

OSCE 4

Instructions for candidate

The brother of one of your patients who has been diagnosed with schizophrenia wants to meet you to discuss his brother's illness, treatment and prognosis. You have only recently joined the team and have limited information about the patient. You do know that this is his first admission to hospital. He had a number of first-rank symptoms of schizophrenia, which improved after several weeks of antipsychotic medication. The patient has given his consent for you to discuss any aspects of his presentation with his brother.

Instructions for actor

Your 23-year-old brother was recently admitted to a psychiatric unit under the Mental Health Act. He left university in his final year without taking his exams. He has since been living at home with you and your 17-year-old sister. Your parents have both died (your mother committed suicide).

Over the past few months your brother has become increasingly withdrawn and isolated. He spends much of his time alone in his room on the Internet. He does go out occasionally with his one remaining friend. However, you suspect that this friend supplies him with cannabis.

In the weeks leading up to his admission your brother started behaving in an increasingly unusual manner. He became aggressive towards his sister and hit her on two occasions. On the day of his admission he was picked up by the police while trying to break into a neighbour's car. He had told you he was increasingly worried that your neighbours were trying to spy on him and were secretly following him every time he went out. The police brought your brother to hospital as they believed he was mentally unwell. He was then admitted for 28 days.

Your brother has improved following admission and will soon be discharged. You now want to know what caused his illness, the nature of the illness and whether, now that he is better, it is likely that he will become ill again.

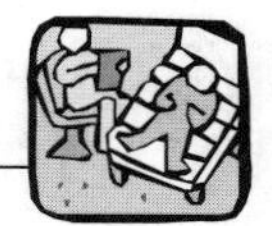

Construct

This OSCE assesses the candidate's ability to communicate effectively and appropriately with a concerned relative. The candidate should be able to answer the relative's questions about his brother's illness, including its aetiology and course.

Examiner's marking sheet

	Excellent	Good	Satisfactory	Fail	Poor
Communication skills					
Discussion of the nature of the illness					
Discussion of the aetiology					
Discussion of the prognosis					
Overall mark					

Communication skills

This OSCE assesses the candidate's ability to establish rapport with a concerned relative. You have been briefed that you are relatively new to the team. This allows you to elicit relevant information from the relative to guide your answers to questions on the aetiology and prognosis. This information should of course be elicited in a sensitive manner.

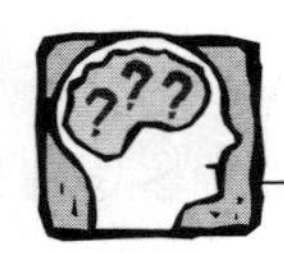

Discussion of the nature of the illness

The primary task under this heading is to explain the main features of the illness. To score maximum marks in this section, your answer should be tailored to the actor's requests. A good way to achieve this is simply to ask 'What would you like to know about.... In response to this questions, the actor may reveal their specific brief for this OSCE.

Be guided by the actor as to how much detail you should provide when describing the illness. A basic explanation of schizophrenia should include its classification as a mental disorder. The disorder includes a number of symptoms which may affect the patient's ability to think clearly or to accurately perceive events occurring in his environment. These symptoms may lead him to reach incorrect conclusions about what is happening to him, and may affect his behaviour. Episodes of illness may recur, but can be treated by a combination of medication and psychological and social approaches.

Once you have provided a basic answer, the actor may then ask more specific questions, or he may move on to other parts of the OSCE as described.

Discussion of the aetiology

Discussion of the aetiology of any presentation should include the addressing of the following relevant factors (the three Ps):

1 **p**redisposing factors

2 **p**recipitating factors

3 **p**erpetuating factors.

You have only been provided with basic information about the patient in your brief. You will therefore need to elicit relevant information from the actor by questioning him further. For example:

> 'The causes of each presentation of schizophrenia are individual for each person.
>
> To try and determine what factors may have specifically contributed to your brother's illness, may I ask you some further questions about his history?'

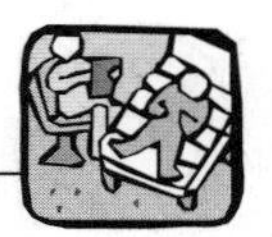

Using this approach, you may elicit that the patient has a probable family history of mental illness and that he was taking cannabis prior to admission.

You should then provide a general description of the aetiology of schizophrenia as being multifactorial. Highlight the fact that there is some evidence that genetic predisposition may play a part (do this sensitively, and be aware that the actor may then ask you about his risk of developing the illness). Also mention that adverse events during childhood may be important, as well as the abuse of certain illicit drugs.

Discussion of the prognosis

Again, to score maximum marks you need to relate the prognosis to the patient's specific history that you have elicited.

You can provide general advice on prognosis, namely that a proportion of patients may never experience another episode of illness, while the remainder may experience either an episodic course or a continuing course.

It is important to try to demonstrate a positive approach which instills a degree of hope in the relative that his brother will not be continuously unwell and distressed. Of course you must be honest and accurate when providing this information, but you should adopt an empathetic approach and highlight the positive prognostic factors. These would include the patient's response to treatment, the relatively short duration of untreated psychosis, and the presence of a precipitant (substance misuse).

Explain to the relative that the prognosis can be improved by efforts to maximise his brother's insight and therefore his compliance with management. Specific help with addressing his cannabis misuse may also improve his prognosis.

OSCE 5

Instructions for candidate

This inpatient has severe depression, which has not responded to two different antidepressants at maximum tolerable doses. During the ward round, electroconvulsive therapy (ECT) has been suggested to the patient by the consultant. Provide the patient with further information on ECT and answer any questions that he has about the risks and benefits of this treatment. The patient has already expressed fears about memory loss.

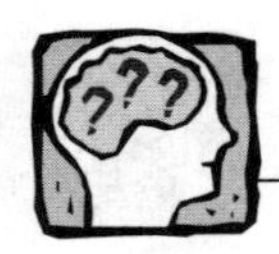

Instructions for actor

You are a 60-year-old man who has had several episodes of depression in the past. Previously your depression has always improved with antidepressant medication.

On this occasion you developed depression after retiring last year from your job as a postman. You have tried two different antidepressants at high doses, but your depression has not improved. Your wife arranged for you to be admitted as you were barely eating or drinking and were at risk of becoming dehydrated.

You remain very depressed with poor appetite, poor sleep, and low levels of energy and concentration. You feel hopeless about your future.

You have been advised that ECT could help your depression. You know little about this treatment, but have seen its depiction in films as being brutal. You also once read that ECT causes permanent brain damage and memory loss. You generally trust the judgement of your psychiatrist, but on this occasion you want more information about ECT before you make a decision.

One of the symptoms of depression is poor concentration. Therefore if the candidate's answer is too long-winded or excessively detailed, ask them to repeat the information because of your concentration problems.

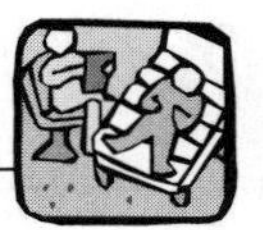

Construct

This OSCE assesses the candidate's ability to explain to a patient with severe depression the benefits and risks associated with ECT. The candidate needs to take into account the fact that the patient has poor concentration and may not be able to follow long or detailed information.

Examiner's marking sheet

	Excellent	Good	Satisfactory	Fail	Poor
Communication skills					
Description of ECT					
Discussion of the benefits of ECT					
Discussion of the risks of ECT					
Overall mark					

Communication skills

In this OSCE you will need to demonstrate an appropriate approach to the patient's concerns about a treatment of which they have limited knowledge. Be aware that in any OSCE which requires the discussion of ECT, the actor may have been briefed to take a negative or even hostile approach to the treatment. This is the case with this OSCE, and you will need to demonstrate to the examiner that you are able to exhibit empathy while addressing the patient's concerns.

You will also need to adapt your answers to take into account the fact that the patient is depressed and has poor concentration. The actor has been briefed not to respond to long-winded or excessively detailed answers. You should be aware that this may happen if you are asked to see a depressed patient in an OSCE. Modify your answers accordingly and remember to use pauses appropriately. If in doubt, ask the patient to repeat your answers or check that they have understood what you have said. Also state that the patient will be given the opportunity to think further about the information you are about to give them. Encourage them to discuss it further with relatives if this would be helpful.

Description of ECT

The description of ECT needs to made carefully to minimise an antagonistic response from the actor. Terms such as 'shock therapy' are probably best avoided. ECT should be defined as standing for 'electroconvulsive therapy', a medical term for a specific form of treatment for severe depression. Then go on to describe ECT. An example of its description is now given.

ECT is a very well-established and safe treatment for depression. It is performed with two doctors present – the treating psychiatrist and an anaesthetist. ECT involves being given a general anaesthetic. The administration of the general anaesthetic is similar to that for a minor operation, consisting of an injection to induce sleepiness and to relax the muscles. This is then followed by inhalation of an anaesthetic gas to keep the patient asleep for several minutes while ECT is applied.

While the patient is under anaesthetic, a small electric current is passed across the brain. This produces a seizure, which is modified by the muscle relaxant. As a result of the small seizure, the chemicals involved in depression are realigned, thus resulting in improved mood. ECT is given twice a week. Usually there is evidence of improved mood after two to four applications. A course of ECT usually consists of 6 to 12 applications, with a review after each treatment.

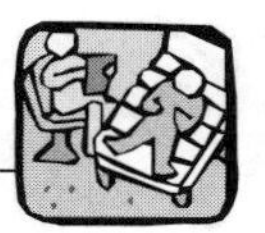

Discussion of the benefits of ECT

As already stated, you should explain that ECT is an established treatment for depression. Studies have shown its usefulness in depression, particularly in severe depression which has not improved in response to antidepressants. Compared with antidepressants, ECT often leads to a more rapid improvement in depression – within 1 to 2 weeks rather than 2 to 4 weeks.

Discussion of the risks of ECT

You should explain that the main serious risk with ECT is actually due to the administration of the general anaesthetic. The risk of death from a general anaesthetic is around 1 in 100 000. To minimise this risk, prior to ECT being performed the patient will undergo a physical examination, blood tests, an ECG and chest X-ray if indicated. The anaesthetist will also conduct a physical review to assess whether the patient is fit to have a general anaesthetic.

You should explain that the main contraindication to ECT is increased pressure within the brain, and that this will be excluded before any ECT is administered.

The actor has been briefed to ask about memory deficits and brain damage resulting from ECT. You should explain that after waking from the anaesthetic, some patients may have a mild headache which can be treated with painkillers. Some patients also experience some disorientation during the initial hours after coming round from the general anaesthetic. Attempts will be made to minimise this by having a dedicated recovery unit, staffed by nurses with expertise in helping patients to wake up from an anaesthetic.

To answer the question on long-term memory problems/brain damage, initially elicit how much the patient knows and what their specific fears may be. Explain that a number of long-term studies have been carried out in patients who have undergone ECT, to determine whether they experience long-term memory problems.

Explain that there is no conclusive evidence to prove that ECT does cause long-term memory problems, other than the memory deficits which occur in the first few hours after the general anaesthetic. Remember to explain that depression often gives the impression of declining memory, as it impairs concentration and thus registration. Therefore as a result of ECT to improve depression, the patient may actually find that remembering things becomes easier rather than more difficult.

A final point to make is that although the majority (80%) of cases improve, not all patients do respond to ECT.

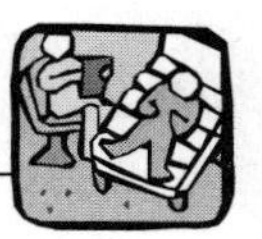

OSCE 6

Instructions for candidate

This patient has just been diagnosed with terminal lung cancer. He has capacity and is not mentally ill. He is refusing any further medical interventions, as he is upset and just wants to go home. The physician looking after the patient has asked you to explain the stages of coming to terms with a terminal diagnosis, so that the patient may be more likely to accept palliative interventions.

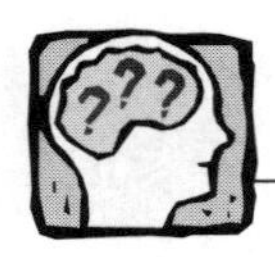

Instructions for actor

You are a 50-year-old male inpatient on a medical ward. You are a lifelong smoker and have been increasingly unwell for several months. You have experienced poor appetite and weight loss. You have had a persistent cough for some time, but have now started to cough up blood. During this admission you have been diagnosed with lung cancer and advised that the cancer is too advanced to be removed.

You are angry that the cancer was not detected sooner, as you went to your GP several weeks ago complaining of a cough. You are now angry with all doctors and cannot see the point in staying in hospital any longer, as your cancer is not treatable.

You have agreed to meet a liaison psychiatrist as you have been informed that they would help to give you a better understanding of what lies ahead. You are somewhat sceptical, but agree to meet the psychiatrist. You are not mentally unwell.

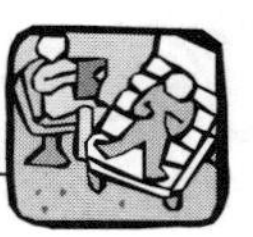

Construct

This OSCE assesses the candidate's ability to communicate with a distressed patient who has received a terminal diagnosis. The candidate should be able to demonstrate empathy, as well as helping the patient to understand the process of coming to terms with a terminal illness. By doing this the candidate should be able to describe the purpose of palliative care.

Examiner's marking sheet

	Excellent	Good	Satisfactory	Fail	Poor
Communication skills					
Discussion of terminal illness					
Discussion of palliative care					
Overall mark					

Communication skills

You have been asked to meet with an angry, distressed patient who has just been told that he is terminally ill. Communication is a major part of this OSCE, and you should allow adequate time to build rapport.

The actor has been briefed to show anger. You should deal with this appropriately, allowing him to ventilate his feelings of anger before continuing with your task.

In every OSCE you should explain who you are and why you are seeing the patient. It would be particularly important to explain this to the present patient. He is on a general medical ward and unless you explain that you are a liaison psychiatrist, he may well at some point ask why you are seeing him.

Discussion of terminal illness

The first task is to establish the extent of the patient's understanding of his terminal diagnosis. You have been told that he has capacity. However, you should confirm with him what he has been told. This will also give him the opportunity to express his feelings and raise any questions that he may have.

Once the diagnosis of a terminal illness has been established, it will be important to show empathy and understanding.

Like all OSCEs, the scenario and task are contrived and have to be performed in seven minutes. In a real clinical situation you would of course spend considerable time building rapport and answering questions. You might want to visit the patient on a number of occasions. However, the task of this OSCE is to demonstrate to the examiner that you are aware of the stages of coming to terms with a terminal diagnosis. You therefore need to explain sensitively to the patient the stages involved.

You should mention that the patient's reaction to receiving such upsetting news is not unusual. Explain that there are still hopefully many months ahead for him, and that the team will try to help him to make the most of his remaining time. Describe to the patient how, to try and achieve this, it is sometimes helpful to understand how people react to such news.

Explain that the initial stage often involves denial of the diagnosis, as it is too distressing to contemplate the news. People sometimes get angry – with their doctor, with themselves, or with God – and ask 'Why did this happen to me?'. They may then bargain for more time.

Sometimes people get stuck in one of these stages, which can result in their last few months being even more distressing. However, by being willing to receive appropriate help and support from professionals, some people reach a position of acceptance and are able to make the most of their remaining time.

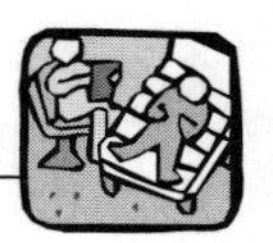

Discussion of palliative care

Again the first task is to establish the patient's understanding of palliative care. The actor has been briefed to say that there is no point in having any further medical contact, as he is going to die.

You should describe the purpose of palliative care as trying to optimise the patient's remaining time. You should state that palliative care involves a multidisciplinary approach. This will include medication for pain relief, appropriate nursing care and psychological support to help him reach acceptance as just outlined.

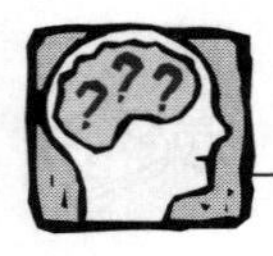

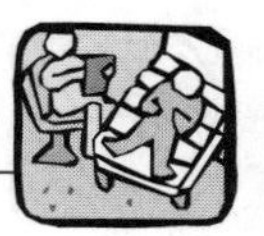

OSCE 7

Instructions for candidate

Assess this patient's attitude and motivation to stop drinking alcohol.

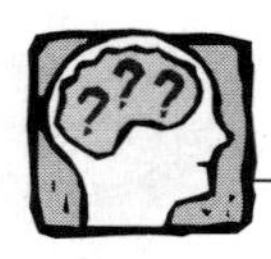

Instructions for actor

You are a 56-year-old divorced woman. You recently lost your job as a secretary after taking long periods of sick leave. From your twenties onwards you have been a very nervous individual, particularly in social settings. You found that alcohol helped to calm your nerves on such occasions and gave you more confidence.

In your thirties your marriage came to an end. To deal with the stress of breaking up with your husband, you started drinking more frequently. Over the past few years your alcohol intake has increased steadily, to the extent that you now drink daily from midday onwards. If you do not drink from midday you start feeling very uncomfortable and shaky and you crave a drink. Having a drink relieves these symptoms.

Whereas originally you would enjoy a variety of different drinks, now you just drink cheap white wine, usually two bottles a day. Once you start drinking you cannot stop, and you drink steadily through the day until you go to bed and collapse.

You have now decided that you must stop drinking. You believe that you are addicted to alcohol and have been feeling depressed for many months. Your children are upset that their mother just spends each day drinking. You have lost both your social life and your job. You fear that your health will suffer as your GP has warned you that your liver cannot cope for much longer. Your GP has referred you to an alcohol service to meet with a psychiatrist to discuss your treatment options.

You have never tried stopping alcohol before and are scared about how difficult this will be for you. Ideally you want to continue enjoying the occasional drink several times a week once you have had treatment.

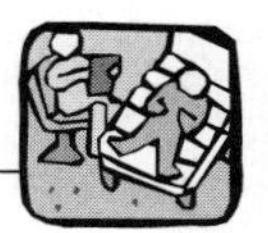

Construct

This OSCE tests the candidate's ability both to establish that the patient is dependent on alcohol and to assess the patient's attitude to their alcohol consumption and their motivation to stop drinking.

Examiner's marking sheet

	Excellent	Good	Satisfactory	Fail	Poor
Communication skills					
Taking an accurate alcohol history					
Establishing the presence of alcohol dependence					
Assessment of attitude to alcohol consumption					
Assessment of motivation to change					
Overall mark					

Communication skills

In an OSCE where you are asked to assess a patient's attitude and motivation to change, it is of course important to demonstrate empathy and a non-judgemental approach.

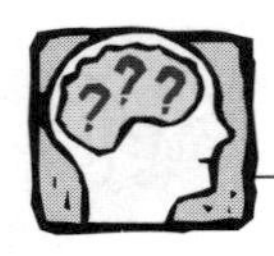

Taking an accurate alcohol history

You will need to demonstrate that you can calculate alcohol consumption correctly (see OSCE 1 for more details on this).

Establishing the presence of alcohol dependence

In this OSCE you will need to assess whether alcohol is problematic for the patient before you can start either to assess her motivation to change or to discuss the treatment options. Using ICD-10 criteria, you should determine whether the patient fulfils the criteria for a disorder due to alcohol.

The most likely diagnoses for an OSCE addressing potentially problematic alcohol usage will be either dependence (see OSCE 1 for details) or harmful use. Harmful use is diagnosed when actual harm has been caused to the patient as a result of drinking, but there is not enough evidence to allow a diagnosis of dependency. In this OSCE you should be able to elicit sufficient information to diagnose alcohol dependence.

Assessment of attitude to alcohol consumption

You will have already partially assessed this by eliciting the pattern of alcohol consumption and confirming dependency. To specifically assess attitude to consumption, you will need to focus in particular on assessing the prominence of drink-seeking behaviour.

Therefore you should spend some time gauging the patient's views on the link between her alcohol consumption and the effects on her marriage, her children, her employment and her social life. Try to identify whether she makes any links between her use of alcohol and the adverse events that have occurred in each of these areas.

The actor has been briefed to state that they accept that alcohol has been deleterious to their mental and physical health. Make sure that you elicit this, as it will help with the next section.

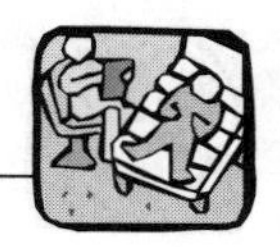

Assessment of motivation to change

You should have established that the patient accepts that alcohol is harming them and that they need to address their intake. Reinforce this by making a comment such as:

> 'You have told me that, because of your drinking, you think you have become depressed and are worried about the state of your liver. You are therefore asking for help to address your alcohol use.'

To try to determine the patient's motivation to change further, ask them what they are willing to do. In particular ask about their views on abstinence and on controlled drinking. As the patient has established alcohol dependence, abstinence would be the preferred option – check whether the patient would be prepared to consider this.

The actor has been briefed to say that they want to carry on drinking eventually, but in lesser amounts. One way to deal with this response is to advise that abstinence would be preferable, as individuals with dependency find it very difficult to achieve controlled drinking. However, you should state that you will support the patient's choice of what to do next. Therefore if they wish to try controlled drinking, advise them that a given period of time can be allowed to try this, but that should controlled drinking lead to reinstatement, they should then consider abstinence.

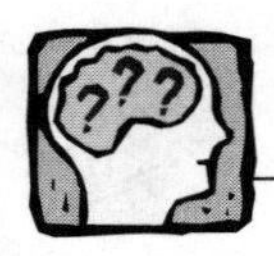

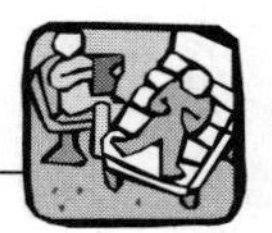

OSCE 8

Instructions for candidate

Confirm to this patient that his distressing physical symptoms are due to panic attacks. He has a family history of ischaemic heart disease (his relatives died at young ages). Address the patient's concerns, explain the nature of his symptoms and discuss the treatment options.

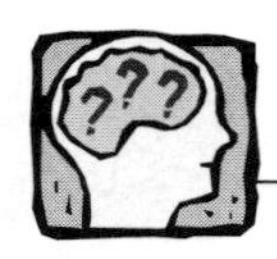

Instructions for actor

You are a 35-year-old man. You went to see your GP complaining that you had experienced several episodes of feeling very unwell, and even fearing that you were about to die.

The first time this happened you became short of breath, had an uncomfortable feeling in your chest, and you became sweaty, nauseous and shaky. Your heart was racing and you thought you were having a heart attack. You asked a passer-by to call an ambulance, which took you to hospital. In hospital the doctor examined you, performed blood tests and took a tracing of your heart. She then stated that your heart was fine and that she could find no serious physical abnormalities.

Initially you were relieved, but you have since experienced more and more of these episodes. Each time you have the same symptoms and feel as if you will either collapse or die. The episodes resolve by themselves after a few minutes, without seeming to result in any physical harm. However, you find it difficult to be reassured, as your father and uncle both died in their fifties from heart attacks. You know that they had similar symptoms to the ones you experience during your episodes.

You are therefore surprised when your GP suggests that you see a psychiatrist about these episodes, which he has termed 'panic attacks'. Reluctantly you visit the psychiatrist at the clinic.

You want to know how the doctors can be sure that there is nothing wrong with you physically. You also wish to know why you are seeing a psychiatrist. Does your GP think you are crazy or inventing these episodes? If these episodes are panic attacks, what are these attacks and why are you experiencing them? Can they be treated effectively?

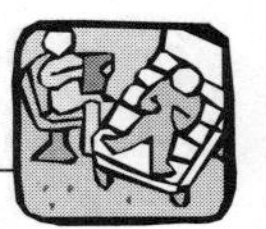

Construct

This OSCE assesses the candidate's ability to explain panic disorder to a patient with distressing somatic and psychological symptoms. It also assesses their ability to explain the available treatments for panic attacks.

Examiner's marking sheet

	Excellent	Good	Satisfactory	Fail	Poor
Communication skills					
Establishing that the symptoms are due to panic attacks					
Explanation of the nature of panic attacks					
Explanation of the available treatments					
Overall mark					

Communication skills

The main communication tasks for this OSCE are to reassure the patient that he is not 'crazy' and to explain to him how psychiatric intervention can help with these episodes. You should elicit that the patient is particularly fearful about the fact that some of his symptoms were experienced by family members who had ischaemic heart disease. You will then be able to compare and contrast his symptoms with genuine symptoms of heart disease.

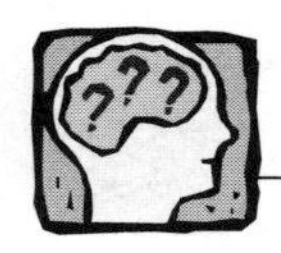

Establishing that the symptoms are due to panic attacks

To establish the diagnosis, you should be able to elicit the main symptoms of panic attacks. The psychological symptoms of panic that this patient experiences are a fear of collapsing or dying. The physical symptoms of panic include dyspnoea, chest discomfort, palpitations, tremor, nausea and sweats.

You should confirm with the patient that he has been reviewed and investigated medically to exclude the presence of a physical cause of these symptoms.

Explanation of the nature of panic attacks

Your main aim will be to explain what panic attacks are and why the patient experiences these particular symptoms.

You should explain that anxiety is a common and appropriate response to threat, and that panic is an extreme anxiety reaction. You could describe how, when a person is threatened or very anxious, their body produces large amounts of adrenaline, rather like someone about to go on stage and deliver a talk.

As a result of these increased levels of adrenaline, a number of symptoms are experienced. These include an increased heart rate, tremor and many of the other symptoms that the patient has experienced. Because individuals in a state of panic experience these symptoms, they jump to the conclusion that they are seriously unwell and something catastrophic is about to happen (eg they may collapse or even die).

Explanation of the available treatments

You should explain that psychiatric intervention can help with these episodes of panic, and that patients are often best helped by a combination of psychological and pharmacological methods.

Explain the psychological approach to treatment, including the use of cognitive behavioural therapy. Include an example of this form of therapy that is relevant to the patient's symptoms. For instance, you could use the example of the patient having believed that he was

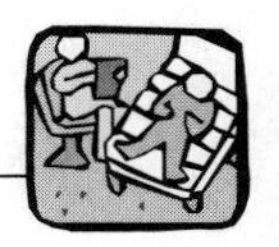

about to die every time he experienced a panic attack, yet he has never suffered any serious physical harm or disability which has persisted beyond the duration of the attack.

You could then explain that cognitive behavioural therapy would look at his thoughts and link them to his experiences, evaluating the evidence for maintaining those beliefs. As a result, the patient may then be able to stop having these catastrophic thoughts during an attack and be able to reassure himself that the attack will soon pass, with no serious adverse outcome.

Finally, you should explain that antidepressant medication can sometimes be useful for lowering overall levels of anxiety. Benzodiazepines such as alprazolam can also have a useful, time-limited role in reducing the number of panic attacks that the patient experiences.

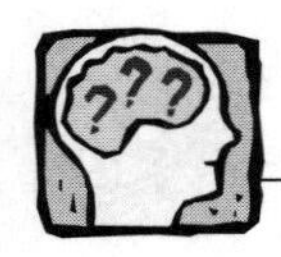

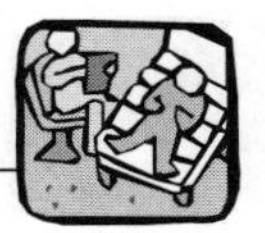

OSCE 9

Instructions for candidate

Take a history from this patient who is attending a follow-up clinic after having recently experienced an episode of depression. Her mood has improved, but she is complaining of continuing loss of libido. Explain the link between depression and sexual dysfunction.

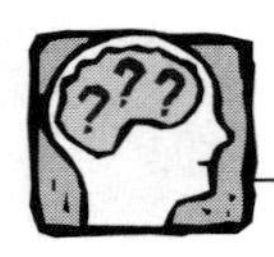

Instructions for actor

You are a 30-year-old nurse who married two years ago. You were referred to a psychiatrist because of problems with depression. This has subsequently improved, but you have persisting problems with sexual dysfunction.

You developed depression eight months ago after a close friend died of cancer. After feeling depressed for several weeks, you found that you could no longer go to work as you felt too drained of energy. Other symptoms that you experienced included poor sleep, waking up early in the morning, poor concentration and loss of sex drive.

You visited your GP, who advised you to start an antidepressant. You did not improve and were referred to a psychiatrist. He gave you some counselling and increased the dose of the antidepressant, and subsequently your depression lifted.

Now you feel that your mood has improved and is almost back to normal. You have returned to work and have started to socialise again. You are visiting the psychiatrist for a follow-up appointment. Your main concern today is that you still have a low sex drive.

You believe the reason for this is that you no longer enjoy sex very much. When you were depressed you lost your sex drive and stopped sleeping with your husband. Since your mood improved, you have resumed having sex but do not find it as enjoyable and cannot reach orgasm (this was not previously a problem).

Your husband is very supportive and you do not feel pressurised about this issue. However, you do have a number of questions. You want to know if your sexual problems are related to the depression. Is the medication contributing to this problem? Will the problem be permanent?

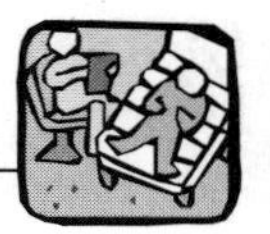

Construct

This OSCE assesses the candidate's ability to establish rapport with a patient who is asking about sensitive personal problems of a sexual nature. The candidate should be able to establish accurately the nature of the sexual dysfunction and its relationship with depression and its treatment.

Examiner's marking sheet

	Excellent	Good	Satisfactory	Fail	Poor
Communication skills					
Establishing the course of the depressive episode					
Establishing the nature of the sexual dysfunction					
Explanation of the link between sexual functioning and depression					
Overall mark					

Communication skills

In this OSCE you are required to ask about sensitive issues of a sexual nature. The actor and examiner are unlikely to be embarrassed by your questions, as they may have played out this scenario many times during the course of the exam. However, you may find it difficult to ask all of the appropriate questions. If this is the case,

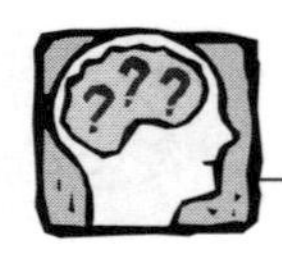

practise OSCEs such as this one with a colleague until you no longer feel embarrassed about asking personal questions.

Establishing the course of the depressive episode

The main tasks of this OSCE are described below. However, you will need to establish that the patient has had her first episode of depression, which was treated with a course of antidepressants.

You will also want to establish that her symptoms have improved, other than those relating to sexual dysfunction.

Establishing the nature of the sexual dysfunction

To score high marks in this section, you will need to demonstrate to the examiner that you have elicited a number of important facts. The best way to do this is to be systematic and use a chronological approach.

The first thing to establish is that the patient had no problems with sexual functioning prior to the onset of depression. After the onset of depression she experienced a loss of libido.

Once the depression had improved, the patient was left with ongoing sexual problems. The main symptom was anorgasmia, which you have established was not previously a problem. If possible, you should try to establish whether this problem started after the onset of antidepressant use. However, it is quite possible that the patient was not having sex around that time because of her depression. It may therefore be difficult to establish precisely a direct link.

The final important point is to ask about the effect that sexual dysfunction is having on the patient's relationship with her husband. In this OSCE, the patient's husband is supportive of her difficulties. This may be important with regard to resolution of this problem.

Explanation of the link between sexual functioning and depression

The patient has presented to you with concerns about the fact that a problem which arose during her depression has remained, despite

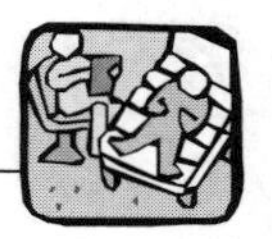

resolution of her other symptoms. You are therefore required to explain to her why this may be so.

You will need to explain that loss of libido is one of the biologically and psychologically mediated symptoms of depression. Once depression improves, sex drive usually returns. The problem with anorgasmia may well be related to the patient's antidepressant.

You should explain that this is the most likely cause, and that it is reversible upon stopping the antidepressant. You should advise taking the pragmatic view that as this is her first episode of depression, the patient should ideally continue with the antidepressant for six months after resolution of the depressive symptoms. As this is a follow-up appointment, the end of that time may be nearing.

After stopping the antidepressant, if the problem remains, the patient can be referred for a specialist opinion to rule out other causes of sexual dysfunction, and for further management.

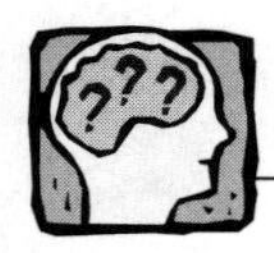

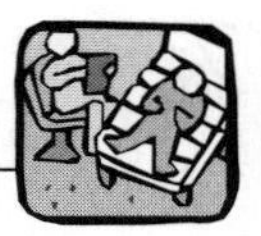

OSCE 10

Instructions for candidate

A 35-year-old married woman is attending clinic, stating that she has stopped taking her lithium therapy. She has had three prior admissions for depression under the Mental Health Act (1983).

One of these admissions followed attempted asphyxiation with car fumes. How would you address the issues and maintain remission?

Instructions for actor

You are a 35-year-old married woman. You have had several episodes of disturbed mood. On occasion your mood has been elevated for days at a time, but you did not require hospital treatment for this as you continued functioning reasonably well. On three occasions you were admitted compulsorily to hospital because of severe depression.

During each admission you were treated with medication, including lithium, which you acknowledge helped improve your mood. However you are unconvinced of the need to take lithium long-term when you are well.

You now wish to become pregnant. You have heard becoming pregnant would be difficult on lithium. You also believe there would be considerable risks of disability to your child if you took lithium during pregnancy. You also want to ask about alternative mood stabilisers.

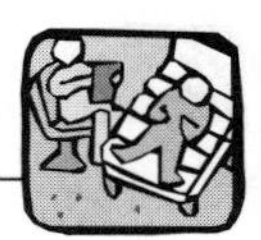

Construct

This OSCE station is primarily testing the candidate's ability to communicate information about treatment succinctly and accurately. It will assess their ability to:

- use appropriate language when discussing non-adherence
- develop a rapport with the patient
- convey essential information, as well as allowing the patient to guide the discussion
- demonstrate knowledge of a common condition and the risks of non-adherence
- discuss alternative treatments.

Examiner's marking sheet

	Excellent	Good	Satisfactory	Fail	Poor
Communication skills					
Explanation of the risks in context					
Discussion of alternatives					
Discussion of outcome and other aspects					
Overall mark					

Communication skills

It is important to establish rapport with the patient and show good use of verbal and non-verbal communication skills. In addition, you need to identify informant concerns and respond to them, and demonstrate an empathetic approach.

Explanation of the risks in context

Make sure that you explain the risks in context, namely that the risk of relapse would be greatly increased, that there would be a significant risk of fetal malformation and that no mood stabiliser is safe in pregnancy.

Lithium is potentially teratogenic, causing cardiac defects and the tetralogy of Fallot. Some studies have estimated the risk of relapse after discontinuation of lithium therapy in patients with bipolar disorder to be 50% within one year. Consequently, it is extremely important to ensure that the patient understands why they need to take the treatment, and how to take it.

Discussion of alternatives

When discussing alternatives, you should mention other antidepressants, psychotherapy and adherence therapy. Adherence therapy involves a mix of behavioural and cognitive approaches.

First, you need to obtain an understanding of the patient's representation of the illness:

- identity – what is it?
- cause – what caused it?
- time-frame – how long will it last?
- consequences – how will it affect or has it already affected the patient?
- cure – can it be controlled or cured?

Behavioural strategies to improve adherence include the following:

- simplification of drug regime
- behavioural prompts
- reinforcement strategies
- rehearsal
- monitoring and diary-keeping.

Cognitive strategies to improve adherence include the following:

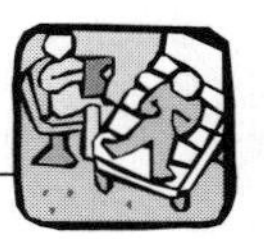

- homework assignments to develop a realistic view of the prognosis
- identifying and replacing inappropriate automatic thoughts with regard to medication and the illness with more appropriate ones
- identifying and developing an action plan to deal with high-risk situations
- reframing or modifying underlying beliefs
- performing a cost-benefit analysis for taking lithium (ie determining the advantages/disadvantages of taking the drug vs the advantages/disadvantages of not taking it).

Other issues to address would include exploring the patient's concerns about taking lithium, the state of her relationship with her partner and why she wishes to stop the medication and start a pregnancy at this particular time.

Discussion of outcome and other aspects

In closing the assessment, the candidate should ensure that there is clarity about which treatment to take, that contraception is being used, and that closer monitoring will take place for a specified period.

Further reading

Moncrieff, J. 1997. Lithium: evidence reconsidered. *British Journal of Psychiatry*, 171, 113–119.

Watkins, E. 2003. Combining cognitive therapy with lithium treatment for bipolar affective disorder. *Advances in Psychiatric Treatment*, 9, 110–115.

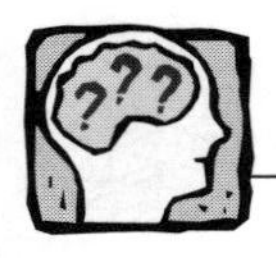

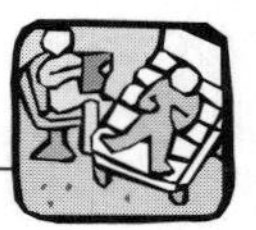

OSCE 11

Instructions for candidate

You have been asked to see a woman who is refusing surgical advice to have her breast cancer treated.

Assess this patient's capacity to refuse treatment.

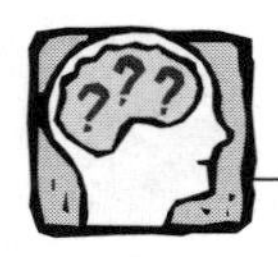

Instructions for actor

You are a 68-year-old housewife. You've been diagnosed with breast cancer which has started to spread. The doctors have discussed treatment options including surgery, radiotherapy, and chemotherapy. You have been advised using all three approaches would mean the five year survival rate would be very high.

However, you do not want to undergo disfiguring surgery.

During the interview the doctor discovers that you do not want to undergo disfiguring surgery ('and how could it be anything else?'). You are worried about your husband's reaction to a wife with breast loss, you are concerned that you would feel 'less of a woman', and you have been told that the treatment might not help anyway.

The radiotherapy caused all your friend's hair to fall out. She was also very ill afterwards and felt sick for a while ('and that was before they started her on chemo'). Then your friend was unable to keep any of her food down.

You feel that you have had a good life, and rather than spending your last years fighting and being unwell you would rather ('just enjoy your family').

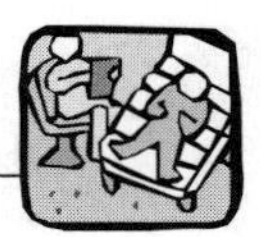

Construct

To pass this OSCE, the candidate must be able to elicit enough information to determine whether the patient has capacity. For this they will need to:

- have an understanding of the requirements for capacity
- determine the patient's beliefs about the illness and treatment
- determine whether the patient is labouring under any defect of reason such that their ability to make decisions is unduly distorted.

Examiner's marking sheet

	Excellent	Good	Satisfactory	Fail	Poor
Communication skills					
Identification of elements of capacity					
Identification of any undue influence					
Overall mark					

Communication skills

It is important to establish a rapport with the patient, to show good use of verbal and non-verbal communication skills, and to demonstrate an empathetic approach.

Identification of elements of capacity and any undue influence

To obtain high marks the candidate must identify the elements of capacity and the information relevant to the decision, determine whether the patient is able to retain the information, and check that the patient can consider the information and reach a decision.

Issues which may need to be addressed include the possibility that there was 'undue influence', the presence of a mental illness, and the fact that the patient does not wish to have chemotherapy or be disfigured (and the reasons for this).

Commentary

In Scotland, relevant legislation in the form of the Adult (Incapacity) Act 2000[1] exists, and in England and Wales there is the Mental Capacity Bill 2004[2]. Common law would only allow an intervention where it is necessary to prevent an immediate risk of harm. The level of risk and the seriousness of the harm must be commensurate with the consequences of the intervention. So intubation of an unconscious patient in respiratory failure would be covered by the 'doctrine of necessity', but vaccination would not. Where the intervention is irreversible the need to demonstrate its necessity increases. So removal of a limb or organ should only occur if no other reasonable option is possible.

Note that if the doctor was aware of a valid advance directive indicating that no intervention was to be allowed under circumstances where the patient was unable to communicate their wishes, the team would be best advised to contact senior colleagues and the legal department immediately, should they wish to proceed against the directive's stated objectives.

Candidates should note that the comment by Lord Justice Butler-Sloss[3] that people must show understanding but not wisdom has been codified in the Bill in paragraph 2(2): 'A person is not to be treated as unable to make a decision merely because he makes an unwise decision.'

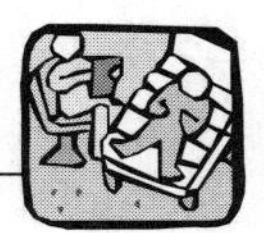

References

1 Adult (Incapacity) Scotland Act 2000.

2 Draft Mental Capacity Bill 2004; www.lcd.gov.uk/menincap/overview.htm

3 *Re T (Adult: Refusal of medical treatment)[1992] All ER 649*

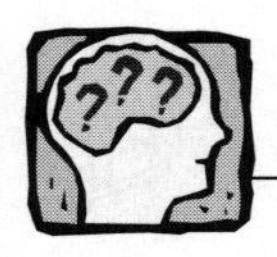

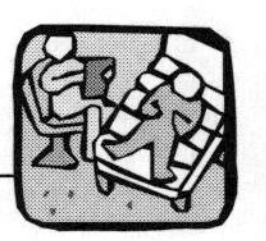

OSCE 12

Instructions for candidate

You have been asked to see an 82-year-old widower on a domiciliary visit. His daughter is a regular visitor and is present when you arrive, but she is due to leave shortly. You have a few minutes to talk with her on the landing outside the flat. Take an appropriate collateral history.

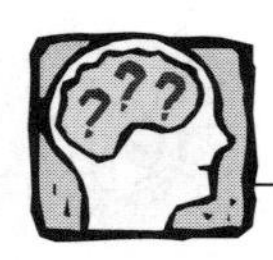

Instructions for actor

You are the middle-aged daughter of a widower of 10 years. You visit your father most days (over a year ago you probably visited once a week). You have noticed that your father is having difficulty shopping, and he dislikes going out as he got lost a while ago. He regularly states that the home help is stealing things. You then find these items around the flat. You are a little upset that he is forgetting the names of his grandchildren, although he has their pictures proudly displayed on the mantelpiece and he still asks after 'the family'.

You have also noticed that he is more emotional than usual, although you could not really say when this began – probably not before you had to increase the frequency of your visits. Last week you found that the kettle had boiled dry, and yesterday the oven was on when you arrived at nine o'clock in the morning. You are not sure whether your father is taking his diabetes tablets properly, as the prescription is lasting for longer than it should. You have not noticed any other changes.

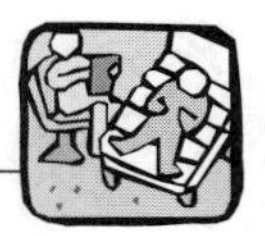

Construct

This OSCE is assessing the candidate's ability to obtain information from a collateral informant. It will test their ability to:

- use appropriate language when assessing a possible case of dementia
- build rapport with the informant
- elicit essential information within a limited time period
- demonstrate a knowledge of the observable elements of dementia.
- assess risk in dementia.

Examiner's marking sheet

	Excellent	Good	Satisfactory	Fail	Poor
Communication skills					
Obtaining an accurate collateral history					
Identifying risk factors					
Overall mark					

Communication skills

This OSCE tests your ability to communicate with a concerned relative. You should demonstrate empathy for the anxieties she has with her father. However you also need to obtain a sufficiently detailed collateral history in order to address the following factors.

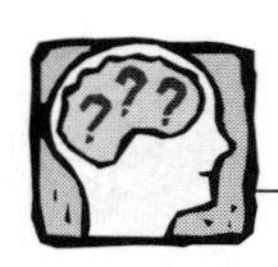

Obtaining an accurate collateral history

The informant may not be able to answer all of your queries with regard to the patient's presentation. This should not stop you asking relevant, important questions.

Areas to focus on include the informant's opinion on the patient's symptoms, such as their memory loss, mood and any somatic symptoms (which may be complicated in the elderly).

Ask about the patient's levels of functioning - in particular any activities of daily living they are no longer able to perform. You should also try and establish any other sources of support.

Identifying risk factors

Try and elicit risk factors from the informant by asking if there have been any recent behaviours which have been of concern and may affect the patient's safety. If the actor has been briefed on such behaviours, then this lead-in question may result in the actor disclosing the specific problem behaviours, rather than you having to ask about every type of risk.

If the actor is not forthcoming, it is important to assess standard risks such as self-harm or violence to others. In addition ask about over or under-medication, food supply (present at home?) and heating/cooking appliances (switched off appropriately?).

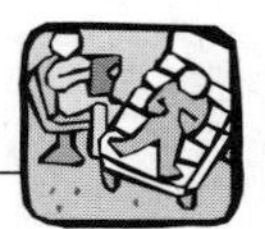

OSCE 13

Instructions for candidate

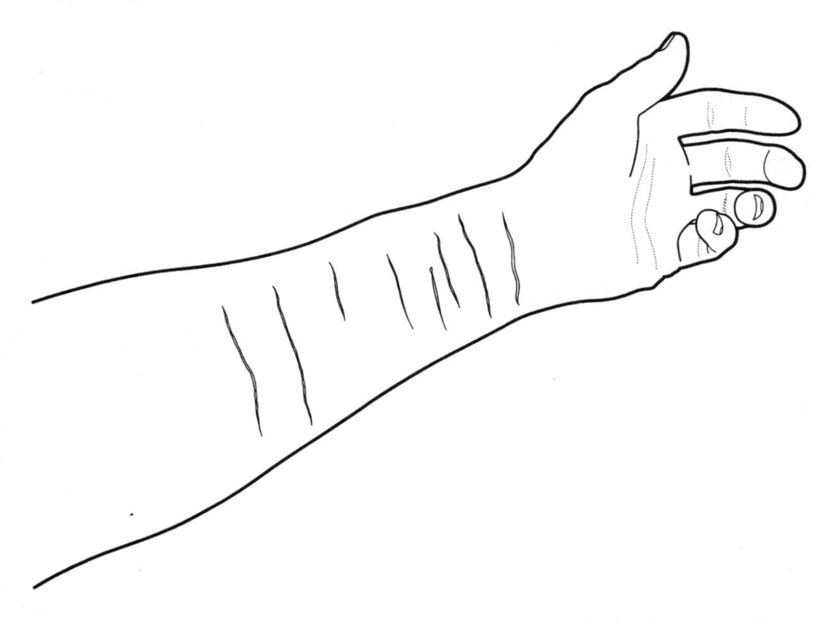

Look at the picture above and then answer the following questions.

1 What is shown in the picture?

2 How are they caused?

3 What is the most likely diagnosis?

4 What (if visible in the above picture) would make you assess the risk as being more severe?

5 What conditions are often comorbid with this diagnosis?

6 What is the likelihood of completed suicide?

Answers to questions

1. Multiple transverse lacerations to the flexor aspects of the forearm(s).
2. Self-inflicted.
3. Personality disorder, unspecified.
4. The presence of any vertical lacerations would greatly increase concerns due to the increased likelihood of severing a deep blood vessel with the resulting raised risk of exsanguination.
5. Other conditions that are frequently present include cluster B personality disorders (dissocial, emotionally unstable and histrionic), depression and substance misuse. Aetiological factors of significance include childhood sexual abuse.
6. The relative risk of completing suicide after an act of deliberate self-harm compared with the normal population over a 10-year period is 100-fold higher.

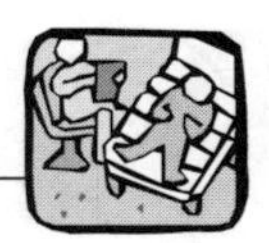

OSCE 14

Instructions for candidate

A 36-year-old woman is referred to you by her GP after her husband has expressed concerns about her eating patterns. Elicit an appropriate history and any other symptoms or behaviours that are relevant.

Instructions for actor

You are a 36-year-old woman who is feeling under increasing pressure to become pregnant. Your feelings about this are markedly ambivalent, and your old patterns of coping under stress are re-emerging.

When you were at university you felt fat and unpopular, so you started to exercise vigorously and to vomit after your lunch. You never lost much weight, as your appetite remained unimpaired, and you enjoyed carbohydrates, such as ice cream and biscuits. You would eat a half-litre tub of ice cream at night when you were feeling tense. Your periods never stopped.

You came to understand as time went on that you were not fat but merely 'above average' weight. As your grades improved and you felt more confident, your comfort eating ceased. You still go to the gym twice a week.

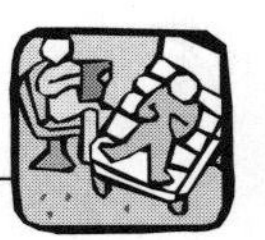

Construct

This OSCE station is primarily assessing the candidate's ability to differentiate between different eating disorders. It will test their ability to:

- develop rapport with the patient
- elicit essential information, as well as allowing the patient to guide the discussion
- demonstrate knowledge of a common area of diagnostic concern.

Examiner's marking sheet

	Excellent	Good	Satisfactory	Fail	Poor
Communication skills					
Assessment of eating history and relevant cognitive factors					
Assessment of associated behaviours and physical symptoms					
Aetiological factors					
Overall mark					

Communication skills

It is important to establish rapport with the patient, to show good use of verbal and non-verbal communication skills, and to demonstrate an empathetic approach.

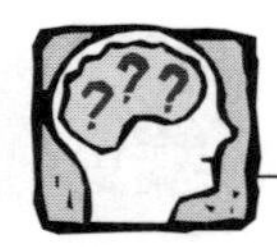

Assessment of eating history and cognitive factors

The following are essential issues:

- eating patterns
- when symptoms started, and changes over time
- previous weight levels
- assessment of quantity/frequency of eating
- reason for dietary habit.

When assessing the cognitive factors, you should attempt to identify any body image disturbance, compulsion to eat or vomit, and associated guilt.

Assessment of associated behaviours and physical symptoms

What are the associated behaviours? Is there bingeing or purging, excessive exercise, or laxative or diuretic use? Are there any physical symptoms (eg menstrual changes, libidinal changes, symptoms of anaemia, muscle weakness/cramps)? What are the patient's height and weight?

Aetiological factors

When you are trying to address aetiology, information about the patient's past history, social circumstances and relationships as well as any other stressors is useful.

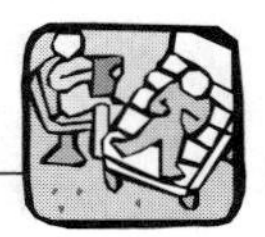

OSCE 15

Instructions for candidate

Review the medication chart below. Comment on any areas of concern and any action that you might take.

<table>
<tr><td colspan="4">Date</td><td></td><td>1/8</td><td></td><td></td><td></td><td></td></tr>
<tr><td colspan="4" rowspan="2">Medication

Ranitidine</td><td>0800</td><td></td><td></td><td></td><td></td><td></td></tr>
<tr><td>1300</td><td></td><td></td><td></td><td></td><td></td></tr>
<tr><td rowspan="2">Route
O</td><td rowspan="2">Fq
OD</td><td rowspan="2">Start date
1/08/04</td><td rowspan="2">Dose
800 mg</td><td>1800</td><td></td><td></td><td></td><td></td><td></td></tr>
<tr><td>(2200)</td><td></td><td></td><td></td><td></td><td></td></tr>
<tr><td colspan="4" rowspan="2">Medication

Risperidone</td><td>(0800)</td><td></td><td></td><td></td><td></td><td></td></tr>
<tr><td>1300</td><td></td><td></td><td></td><td></td><td></td></tr>
<tr><td rowspan="2">Route
O</td><td rowspan="2">Fq
BD</td><td rowspan="2">Start date
1/08/04</td><td rowspan="2">Dose
2 mg</td><td>1800</td><td></td><td></td><td></td><td></td><td></td></tr>
<tr><td>(2200)</td><td></td><td></td><td></td><td></td><td></td></tr>
<tr><td colspan="4" rowspan="2">Medication

Chlorpromazine</td><td>0800</td><td></td><td></td><td></td><td></td><td></td></tr>
<tr><td>1300</td><td></td><td></td><td></td><td></td><td></td></tr>
<tr><td rowspan="2">Route
O</td><td rowspan="2">Fq
Nocte</td><td rowspan="2">Start date
1/08/04</td><td rowspan="2">Dose
50 mg</td><td>1800</td><td></td><td></td><td></td><td></td><td></td></tr>
<tr><td>(2200)</td><td></td><td></td><td></td><td></td><td></td></tr>
<tr><td colspan="4" rowspan="2">Medication

Zopiclone</td><td>0800</td><td></td><td></td><td></td><td></td><td></td></tr>
<tr><td>1300</td><td></td><td></td><td></td><td></td><td></td></tr>
<tr><td rowspan="2">Route
O</td><td rowspan="2">Fq
Nocte</td><td rowspan="2">Start date
1/06/04</td><td rowspan="2">Dose
15 mg</td><td>1800</td><td></td><td></td><td></td><td></td><td></td></tr>
<tr><td>(2200)</td><td></td><td></td><td></td><td></td><td></td></tr>
</table>

To gain the most from this question write your answers down before proceeding.

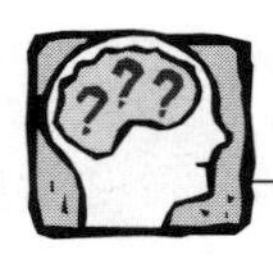

Scoring guide

A candidate who covers the following areas of concern will score well:

1 Risperidone is being prescribed as a BD (twice a day) regime. Why is this? Its half-life allows once daily dosing. Twice daily dosing increases the risk of poor compliance.

2 The patient has been on a high dose (15 mg) of Zopiclone, a hypnotic, for more than 28 days. This drug is not licensed for long-term use; there is evidence of addictive potential. The CSM wrote on this issue in Spring 2004. The licensed indication is for 3.75–7.5 mg.

3 The patient is also receiving chlorpromazine at night. If this drug is being used as an adjunct to the Zopiclone, what other steps have been considered? If it is being used as an antipsychotic, why is there polypharmacy? The National Service Framework: Schizophrenia National Institute for Clinical Excellence 2002 guidelines on the treatment of schizophrenia indicate that monotherapy should be the norm.

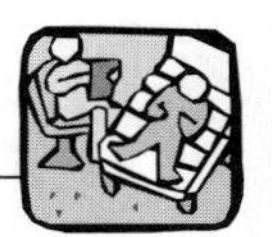

OSCE 16

Instructions for candidate

This is the medication chart for a 54-year-old woman with newly diagnosed rheumatoid arthritis. What questions does it raise? Consider what problems may emerge and how you would manage them.

Date					1/8	2/8	3/8	4/8	5/8	6/8	7/8	8/8	9/8	10/8
Medication				0800										
Lithium carbonate (Priadel)				1300										
Route O	Fq OD	Start date 1/08/03	Dose 800 mg	1800										
				2200	IA	IA	IA	IA	IA	IA	STOP			
Medication				0800										
Lithium citrate (Priadel) 520 mg/5 mL				1300										
Route O	Fq OD	Start date 7/08/03	Dose 20 mL	1800										
				2200							IA	IA	IA	
Medication				0800	PD	PD	PD	PD	PD	PD	PD	PD	PD	PD
Ibuprofen				1300										
Route O	Fq BD	Start date 10/08/03	Dose 0.8 g	1800										
				2200	IA	IA	IA	IA	IA	IA	IA	IA	IA	
Medication				0800										
Fybogel				1300										
Route O	Fq OD	Start date 10/08/03	Dose 1 sachet	1800										
				2200	IA	IA	IA	IA	IA	IA	IA	IA	IA	

To gain the most from this question write your answers down before proceeding.

Scoring guide

A candidate who covers the following areas of concern will pass:

- Why was this patient's medication changed from one preparation of lithium to another? Was it medication error, or some other reason? The two preparations are not bio-equivalent: Despite the brand being identical! 200mg of lithium carbonate is the equivalent to 509 mg of lithium citrate.
- While this change may be legitimate it would require the same degree of monitoring as an initiation of treatment. She will therefore require weekly levels of her trough lithium plasma concentration for at least four weeks. However, generally after five to seven weeks the levels increase, typically from 0.8 to 1.0 mmol/L. Thereafter plasma levels are required monthly for three months, then three-monthly.
- Unfortunately this lady also has rheumatoid arthritis. NSAIDs can raise plasma lithium levels. So there will need to be even more caution which will need to be maintained as her anti-inflammatory treatment is altered.
- Renal tubular clearance of lithium is inhibited by the prostaglandin pathways in the kidney, an unavoidable effect when NSAID's are used, for their anti-inflammatory and analgesic actions.

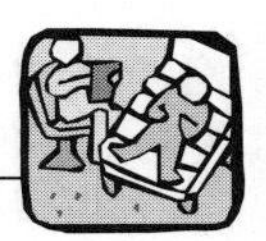

OSCE 17

Instructions for candidate

You have assessed Mr B, aged 47 years, in the outpatient clinic. He has been experiencing intrusive memories and vivid dreams following an incident in which he was threatened with a chainsaw by a workman. He repeatedly sees, in his mind's eye, 'his teeth flying across the garden' and 'gore splattering everywhere'. He is reluctant to go out as he does not wish to bump into the assailant. The police are not pursuing the matter. Mr B startles easily, finds that he is always aware of any building work that is going on, and has been terrified of loud noises since the incident occurred three months ago. Discuss with Mr B his queries about psychological treatment for his symptoms.

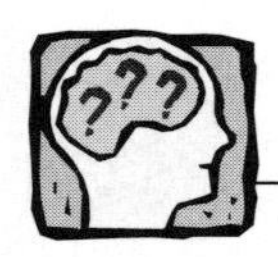

Instructions for actor

You are a 47-year-old man attending clinic. Several months ago you confronted a workman outside your home as he was throwing debris onto your lawn. The workman became verbally aggressive towards you. When you attempted to stand up to him, he threatened you with the chainsaw he was holding. You genuinely felt he was going to seriously injure you and you fled inside your home.

Since then you have persistently relived the experience mentally. You have flashbacks of the episode, accompanied by unpleasant fantasies of what would have happened to you, had the workman attacked you with the chainsaw. You also have nightmares about this episode. You are now always fearful when approaching building sites and sudden loud noises terrify you.

You have been seen in clinic previously and diagnosed with post-traumatic stress disorder (PTSD). You were advised to take medication, but you are reluctant to take pills. You would prefer a 'talking' treatment.

You have looked up PTSD on the internet and come across a promising treatment called EMDR - eye movement desensitisation and reprocessing. In particular today you want to know what is the treatment, how does it work and how long will it take.

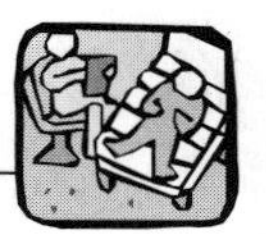

Construct

This OSCE station is primarily assessing the candidate's ability to communicate information about treatment succinctly and accurately. It will test their ability to:

- use appropriate language when discussing a particular therapy
- develop rapport with the patient
- convey essential information, as well as allowing the patient to guide the discussion
- demonstrate knowledge of a common condition
- discuss developing treatments which remain contentious.

Scoresheet

	Excellent	Good	Satisfactory	Fail	Poor
Communication skills					
Establishes diagnosis of PTSD					
Explanation of psychological therapy					
Overall mark					

Communication skills

It is important to establish rapport with the patient and show good use of verbal and non-verbal communication skills. You will need to identify concerns and respond to them, and demonstrate an empathetic approach.

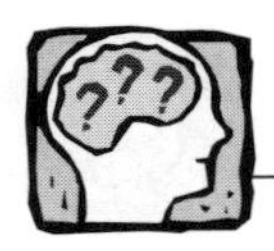

Establishes diagnosis of PTSD

This patient has already received a diagnosis of PTSD. The main task of the OSCE is to discuss psychological treatment of this condition, in particular the use of EMDR. However, you should confirm that the patient does have PTSD by asking about the following criteria:

- Exposure to a traumatic event of sufficient severity to cause pervasive distress in almost anyone
- Persistent reliving of the trauma in the form of intrusive memories or nightmares
- Avoidance of cues which remind the patient of the original trauma
- Autonomic hyperarousal
- Emotional blunting

You should explain that it will be necessary to tolerate high levels of arousal, that pharmacotherapy is not very effective, and that once the proposed treatment has been discontinued the symptoms may return. The technique of eye movement desensitisation and reprocessing (EMDR) depends on a neural circuit that counteracts fear. The process of EMDR overrides fear by linking safe thoughts with the fear-provoking conditioned stimulus. The immediate effects of EMDR are to reduce the patient's arousal levels so that emotional and cognitive processing can occur without automatic inner avoidance.

Explanation of psychological therapy

When explaining the structure of the treatment it would be useful to indicate that:

- it is a 'talking therapy' which is delivered on a one-to-one basis
- sessions are typically held once a week for 5 to 7 weeks
- there will be homework for the patient to do between sessions.

Discussion of outcome

Prognostically the outcome is good, and there is usually a substantial reduction in distress relating to the traumatic memory. However, EMDR will not resolve unrelated issues. Evidence for the efficacy of this treatment includes both psychological measures and differences between pre- and post-treatment imaging studies.

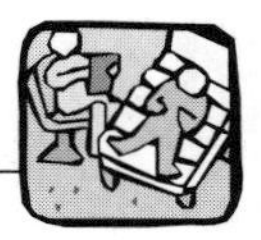

Commentary

EMDR is an eight-stage process that was developed by Shapiro. It involves taking a history, patient preparation, assessment, desensitisation (counter-conditioning), installation of new cognitive processes ('installation'), checking for somatic symptoms ('body scan'), closure and re-evaluation. Although EMDR was initially viewed with scepticism by mainstream psychiatry, further studies on non-heterogeneous populations with post-traumatic stress disorder have shown consistent improvement as a result of treatment. Brain imaging studies have shown changes in cerebral metabolism after treatment. The process is a very carefully controlled exercise involving a thorough evaluation of the patient, including their propensity for dissociation, the role of avoidance in the maintenance of their symptom clusters, and their coping strategies. Before treatment begins the patient is educated about the illness and the EMDR process, and is given training in any skills that may be required to deal with issues which are raised after treatment.

Negative cognitions which may be linked to the trauma are identified and challenged. Rapidly alternating bilateral stimuli are used to reduce the traumatic memories and then install a more appropriate cognition. Once the 'Subjective Unit of Distress' has fallen to minimal levels and the 'Validity of Cognition' of the appropriate cognition has risen to a high level the process is almost complete. The patient 'scans' their body for any residual stress, manifested as any unusual sensations, and once these have been resolved by further bilateral stimuli the process is complete. Further sessions are important for reviewing any unresolved memories that may arise when the level of affect has been reduced and previously blocked experiences may be accessed. In addition, any secondary stimuli may need to be worked on, to prevent reconditioning from occurring.

Further reading

MacCulloch, M.J. 1999. Eye movement desensitisation and reprocessing. *Advances in Psychiatric Treatment*, 5, 120–126.

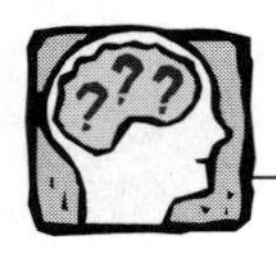

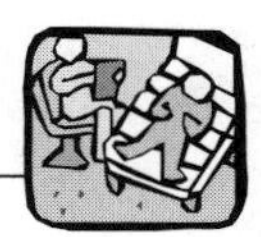

OSCE 18

Instructions for candidate

You have been called to the psychiatry ward by a nurse, who tells you that the father of one of your patients has arrived and is asking to speak to you.

The patient is a 23-year-old man with a first episode of psychosis. He was troubled by paranoid delusions, believing that his life was in danger and carrying a knife with him for protection. He was seen at home one week ago and detained under the Mental Health Act 1983. On admission to hospital he was given haloperidol 10 mg im and lorazepam 4 mg im for severe agitation. The next day he was started on olanzapine 10 mg orally. Yesterday he was transferred to the intensive-care unit suffering from neuroleptic malignant syndrome.

Answer the father's questions about the management of his son's illness.

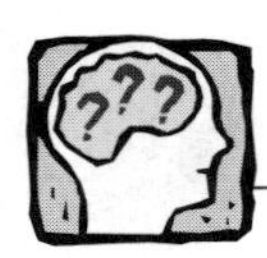

Instructions for actor

You are the father of a 23-year-old man who was recently admitted to the psychiatry ward. You have been told that he has a mental illness and that he requires urgent treatment.

You have noticed a deterioration in your son's health since he returned from a holiday in South-East Asia a year ago. He became moody and less sociable. He spent increasing periods of time in his bedroom, and you and your wife would often hear him talking in his room as if he was having a conversation with another person. He would frequently play loud music, but when confronted about this he would just stare and mumble. His conversation was sometimes difficult to understand, and he was irritable and argumentative. In recent weeks he had taken an increasing interest in news stories about war, often talking about his life being in danger because of what he knew.

You approached your family doctor for advice. He came to see your son and then arranged for him to be seen by a social worker and a psychiatrist. Your son was 'sectioned' despite your protests. However, you were promised that it was in his best interests and he would receive appropriate help in hospital.

Earlier today you were telephoned by the ward staff to be told that your son's condition has deteriorated and he has been transferred to intensive care. You rushed to see him and he seems to be in a very bad way, wired up to monitors and being given fluids by tubes. You are now on the psychiatry ward, waiting to see a doctor and to get some answers about what has happened. You are very angry about the situation, and you ask many challenging questions.

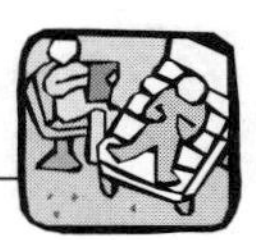

Construct

This OSCE assesses the candidate's ability to control an interview with an angry relative, to demonstrate knowledge of an emergency situation and to communicate details of this emergency condition to a lay person.

Examiner's marking sheet

	Excellent	Good	Satisfactory	Fail	Poor
Communication skills					
Explanation of the aetiology, symptoms and signs of neuroleptic malignant syndrome					
Explanation of the emergency management of neuroleptic malignant syndrome					
Explanation of the future management and prognosis					
Overall mark					

Communication skills

In OSCE stations in which you are asked to talk to a relative, you can expect to be asked many questions and to face a range of emotions.

It is important to listen to the father and allow him to express his anger and distress. He is likely to be feeling guilty about not having done more to prevent his son's admission. Try not to interrupt him, but instead listen patiently and address each of the areas of

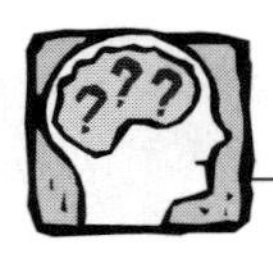

concern. Avoid the use of jargon, and after any explanation you have given, make sure that he has understood you. You should appear authoritative yet empathetic. Acknowledge the distress that the situation has caused to the father. There is no harm in saying you are sorry that his son has taken a turn for the worse.

It is important to adopt an open attitude by not appearing defensive or as if you have something to hide. Do not mislead the father with factual errors. If you do not know the answer to a question, say so.

Explanation of the aetiology, symptoms and signs of neuroleptic malignant syndrome

You need to explain the idiosyncratic nature of neuroleptic malignant syndrome, namely that it can occur with any neuroleptic medication, at any dose and at any time. The incidence is reported to be between 0.1 % and 0.5 %. Therefore it is almost impossible to predict. However, as a doctor you are trained to detect the symptoms and signs of the condition and take appropriate action.

The aetiology of neuroleptic malignant syndrome is not fully understood, but it is related to an underlying neurotransmitter abnormality.

The symptoms of the condition include a raised body temperature, rigidity of muscles and autonomic dysfunction, which may include a fast heart rate, labile blood pressure, sweating, urinary incontinence and pallor.

Explanation of the emergency management of neuroleptic malignant syndrome

Investigations that you may order to confirm your clinical impression normally include blood tests, which may show a raised white cell count, raised creatine phosphokinase levels and abnormalities in the liver function tests.

You need to explain to the patient's father that this is a potentially life-threatening condition, with a mortality rate of 20%. Therefore urgent and intensive medical and nursing care is required, and this is why his son is on an intensive-care ward. The management of the condition includes stopping the neuroleptic medication that is

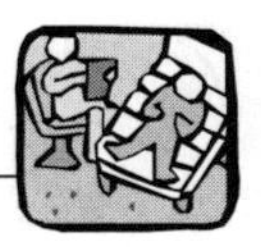

thought to be the cause. Other treatments that have been tried in more severe cases include the use of benzodiazepines, trials of dopamine agonists such as bromocriptine or amantadine, and the use of dantrolene and electroconvulsive therapy.

Explanation of the future management and prognosis

With early recognition and intensive treatment the mortality rate drops to about 5%. If there are no complications, the syndrome lasts for 7 to 10 days in cases that have been receiving oral neuroleptics. As soon as the patient is medically fit, he will return to the psychiatry ward. He may then be treated with an alternative neuroleptic medication, although the same one may be used in some circumstances.

Further reading

Neuroleptic Malignant Syndrome Information Service; www.nmsis.org

Bristow, M.F. and Kohen, D. 1993. How 'malignant' is the neuroleptic malignant syndrome? *British Medical Journal,* 307, 1223–1224.

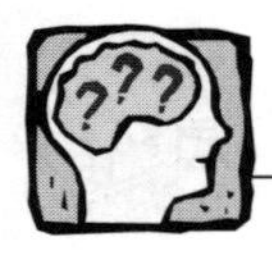

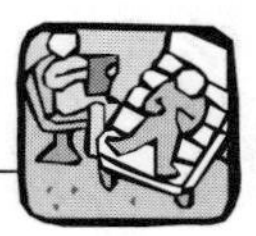

OSCE 19

Instructions for candidate

You are interviewing a 30-year-man who was admitted voluntarily 8 weeks ago with a relapse of a schizophrenic illness. He was first diagnosed with schizophrenia 6 years ago. He has been on a number of oral and depot neuroleptics (both typical and atypical) over the years, and has been hospitalised on three occasions. His present admission was because of auditory hallucinations telling him to kill himself. He cut his wrists with a kitchen knife before he was discovered by a care worker in the residential accommodation in which he was staying.

You need to obtain the patient's informed consent for the initiation of treatment with clozapine.

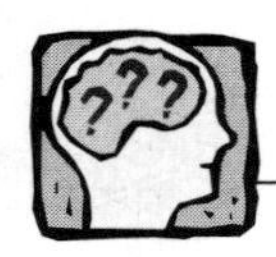

Instructions for actor

You are a 30-year-old man who has been diagnosed with schizophrenia. You are an inpatient on a psychiatry ward to which you were admitted 8 weeks ago.

Your symptoms include hearing voices outside your head telling you to harm yourself or others around you. Usually these voices are controlled by medication, but sometimes they get out of control and you are admitted to hospital so that your treatment can be reviewed. This is what happened this time. You were on a drug called risperidone and living in the community. After you were admitted, this drug was changed to olanzapine. However, this has not helped and you remain unwell.

The doctor has mentioned starting a new drug, which is the reason for this interview.

You want to know more about the treatment that the doctor is proposing. You know that the drug is called clozapine, but not much more. If the doctor says that it is the best drug for you, you will ask why you were not prescribed it earlier.

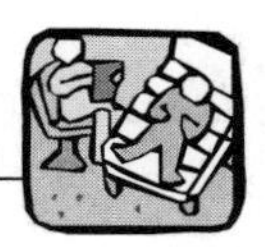

Construct

This OSCE assesses the candidate's knowledge of therapy for treatment-resistant schizophrenia, specifically with clozapine. The candidate should demonstrate obtaining the patient's informed consent.

Examiner's marking sheet

	Excellent	Good	Satisfactory	Fail	Poor
Communication skills					
Description of the rationale for treatment with clozapine					
Explanation of the side-effects of clozapine treatment					
Description of the Clozaril Patient Monitoring Service and the treatment regime					
Overall mark					

Communication skills

Obtaining informed consent for a treatment involves more than just asking the patient whether he agrees to take the treatment that you are proposing.

For the patient, it is a free choice. You must not force him to accept what you wish to prescribe. Make sure that he understands any information you give him, and that you answer any questions he

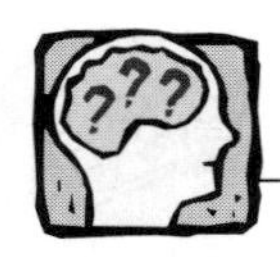

may have. It is important to avoid the use of medical jargon which the patient may not understand.

You must explain that the patient's treatment will not be affected if he does not agree to clozapine treatment, that consent can be withdrawn at any time and that it will be documented in the medical notes. You should also explain to the patient the alternative treatments that are available.

Description of the rationale for treatment with clozapine

In 2002 the National Institute for Clinical Excellence (NICE) published guidance on the use of the newer (atypical) neuroleptic drugs to treat schizophrenia. This guidance stated that in individuals with evidence of treatment-resistant schizophrenia, clozapine should be introduced at the earliest opportunity. Treatment-resistant schizophrenia is suggested by a lack of satisfactory clinical improvement despite the sequential use of the recommended doses of at least two neuroleptics, at least one of which should be an atypical, for six to eight weeks.

If treatment with clozapine is continued for up to one year, improvement is seen in more than 60% of patients.

Explanation of the side-effects of clozapine treatment

The most serious side-effects are neutropenia and agranulocytosis. The latter is potentially fatal, so the use of clozapine is restricted to patients who are registered with the Clozaril Patient Monitoring Service (see below). Clozapine is stopped immediately if there is a fall in the patient's white cell count.

Other side-effects include nausea, vomiting, hypersalivation, sedation, constipation, tachycardia, nocturnal enuresis, benign hyperthermia and elevation of liver enzymes. Long-term treatment may cause weight gain.

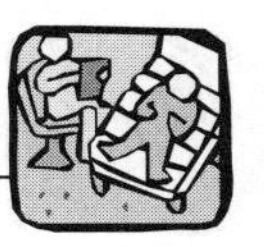

Description of the Clozaril Patient Monitoring Service and the treatment regime

The patient needs to be registered with the Clozaril Patient Monitoring Service (CPMS) before commencement of clozapine treatment. The small risk of neutropenia is detected by regular haematological monitoring through the CPMS. Leukocyte and differential blood counts must be normal before clozapine treatment is started. Counts are monitored every week for 18 weeks, and thereafter at least every four weeks. With periodic blood monitoring, the risk of agranulocytosis is 0.38%.

The patient should be asked to report any signs of infection, such as a sore throat or fever, which may indicate the presence of agranulocytosis. A blood test will be necessary to exclude this possibility.

Clozapine is available as a tablet to be taken by mouth. The dose is titrated upward according to the patient's response and only if blood results are normal. The starting dose is 12.5 mg once or twice on the first day, 25-50 mg on the second day, and then the dose is increased gradually in steps of 25-50 mg over two to three weeks to 300 mg daily in divided doses. If necessary, the daily dose may be increased further. The usual dose is 200-450 mg daily. Above 200 mg, the total daily dose should be divided and a larger portion of the dose may be given at night. The maximum dose is 900 mg daily.

If the patient does not take clozapine for more than two days, the medication is restarted at 12.5 mg once or twice daily on the first day, but it may be feasible to increase the dose more quickly than on initiation.

Further reading

The most recent edition of the *British National Formulary*, published by the British Medical Association and the Royal Pharmaceutical Society of Great Britain.

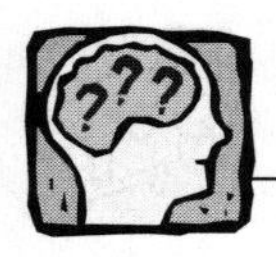

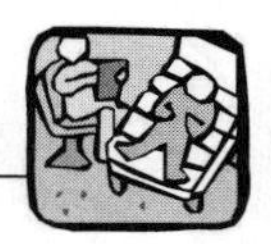

OSCE 20

Instructions for candidate

You have been urgently called to the casualty department of a hospital to see a 39-year-old man who has been brought in by the police. He was detained at Heathrow Airport, London, in the early hours of the morning when he tried to get on a plane to New York without a ticket or passport. When confronted by security staff, he caused a major disturbance, shouting that he was a pilot and that he wanted to take his plane to Monte Carlo.

Assess the risks that this man presents.

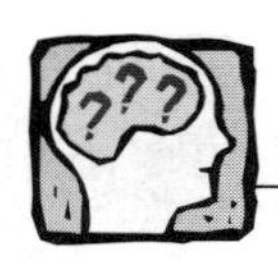

Instructions for actor

You are a 39-year-old man who has suffered from depression since your divorce five years ago. Six weeks ago your family doctor started you on venlafaxine, an antidepressant.

During the last month your behaviour has changed. You feel very happy and are constantly smiling, laughing and telling jokes. You feel extremely energetic and you have been very active. You feel restless and cannot sit down for any length of time. You do not feel hungry, and you may even have lost some weight. You do not feel tired either, despite the fact that you are not sleeping properly.

During the last fortnight you have bought a number of luxury goods on impulse using a credit card, including a designer watch (for £500), a sports car (£2500 deposit) and a television set (for £1500). You gave £250 to a beggar in the street and you donated £500 to a charity event in Scotland that had been publicised on a television programme.

Your libido is raised and your normally introspective nature has given way to more extroverted behaviour. You have chatted up several women in pubs and clubs. In the last week you have visited four prostitutes and had unprotected sex on each occasion.

Today you decided to go to Monte Carlo because you have heard it is the place to gamble. You believe you can pilot the Boeing 737 aeroplane that you apparently own at Heathrow Airport. You went to the airport, but for some reason you were not allowed to go to your plane. You were arrested by the police after you became irritable. You do not know why you are in hospital waiting to see a psychiatrist, because you do not feel depressed.

You appear happy and over-friendly, commenting on the doctor's good-looking features and great dress sense. You try to guess the name of the doctor's aftershave/perfume. You invade their personal space by moving your chair close to theirs. You talk faster than normal and are easily distracted, moving on to irrelevant details quickly. You fidget a lot in your seat, and you may get up and walk around at times.

You do not believe that you are ill. You do not think you need medication – indeed you have stopped your antidepressants now that you are well – nor do you think that you need to be admitted to

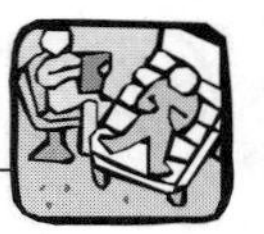

a ward. If the doctor insists on probing any of these points, you become irritable and hostile.

Construct

This OSCE assesses the candidate's ability to carry out a risk assessment on a patient with symptoms of mood elevation. The candidate should be able to illustrate the severity of the condition and gather enough information to justify using the Mental Health Act 1983 to admit the patient.

Examiner's marking sheet

	Excellent	Good	Satisfactory	Fail	Poor
Demonstration of a safe approach to interviewing					
Communication skills					
Eliciting symptoms of mood elevation					
Assessment of risk					
Exploration of possible aetiological factors					
Overall mark					

Demonstration of a safe approach to interviewing

The information that you have been given suggests that the patient is agitated. Show the examiner that you are aware of safety consid-

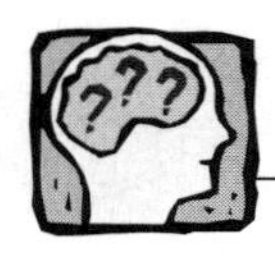

erations by moving the chairs so that you are sitting nearest to the exit, and removing any objects which may be used as weapons.

Communication skills

Do not rush to interrupt the patient so that you can begin your questions. Allowing the patient to speak for a few minutes may illustrate the psychopathology of their condition, such as pressure of speech and flight of ideas. The content of the speech may reveal the symptoms of mania. You should reflect back to the patient what you have heard, to demonstrate to the examiner that you are detecting abnormalities. For example:

> 'I find it difficult to follow your speech because you are jumping between different topics. Have you noticed this, too?'
>
> 'Can you explain to me what happened at the airport? It seems rather bizarre.'

Eliciting symptoms of mood elevation and assessment of risk

There are several symptoms of mania to be elicited, each of which may be putting both the patient and others at risk of harm:

- mood elevation and/or irritability
- increased self-esteem and grandiosity
- increased activity and restlessness
- increased sociability, over-familiarity and talkativeness
- overspending and other reckless and irresponsible behaviour
- increased sexual energy.

Rather than running through a quick checklist of symptoms, you should listen to the patient, pointing out symptoms as he describes them. and then explore those symptoms which he has not talked about. For example:

> 'You say you have bought a watch for £500. That seems an expensive purchase to make on impulse. Have you bought anything else or given money away?'
>
> If a thought seems to be bizarre, explore it further and demonstrate to the examiner whether it is a delusion. For example:

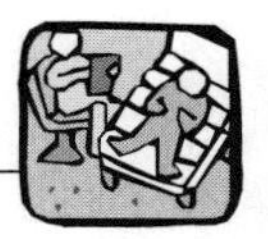

'You say that you are a pilot. How long have you been a pilot? Where did you train? How long is the training period? How could you afford the aeroplane?'

Exploration of possible aetiological factors

Often a good way to determine the cause of an episode of illness is to determine when it started and ask the patient whether he knows the cause. For example:

'So you've been feeling this well for about four weeks. Did anything happen or change in the last month or two that you think has made you feel so good?'

'Has anything like this happened before? What was the cause last time?'

Further reading

Morriss, R. 2004. The early warning symptom intervention for patients with bipolar affective disorder. *Advances in Psychiatric Treatment*, 10, 18-26.

Young, A.H., Macritchie, K.A.N. and Calabrese, J.R. 2000. Treatment of bipolar affective disorder. *British Medical Journal*, 321, 1302-1303.

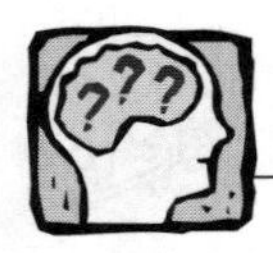

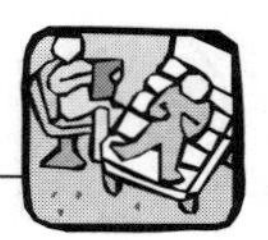

OSCE 21

Instructions for candidate

You are on a medical ward interviewing a man who was admitted three days ago with upper abdominal pain and haematemesis. His blood results show a macrocytic anaemia and abnormal liver function tests. An upper gastrointestinal endoscopy reveals oesophageal varices and acute gastritis.

Take a history to illustrate the complications of alcohol dependency.

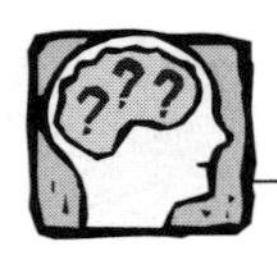

Instructions for actor

You are a 26-year-old man who is divorced and unemployed. You live alone in a rented council flat.

You have had problems with heavy drinking for 8 years. You started drinking when you went to university at the age of 18 years. Three years later, when you started employment as a sales representative, you found it difficult to cope with the stress of achieving monthly sales targets, and you started to drink alcohol regularly. Over a 2-year period your drinking became out of control. You were frequently late for work and your absenteeism rate was high. You were eventually dismissed when you were convicted of drink-driving and given a 12-month driving ban.

You married your girlfriend after you had both graduated from university. At first the marriage was successful. However, as you turned to drink, the relationship deteriorated. You frequently lost your temper with your wife, and you hit her on two occasions. She left you on three occasions before eventually filing for divorce. You have no children from this relationship.

You have been unable to hold down another job and you are no longer in a relationship. You spend any money that you have on alcohol. You are given credit by the local off-licence shop. You have outstanding debts both to the utilities and to two credit card companies. You lost your home last year because you could not keep up the mortgage repayments.

You have been neglecting yourself, and your health has worsened in recent months. You have stomach pains and weight loss. Your mood is low and you have been lacking motivation. Your memory is poor and you find it difficult to concentrate on tasks. You are not sleeping properly and you always feel tired. You frequently think about ending your life, although you have never made any plans. If you do not drink regularly, you get a headache and you notice that your hands shake, you perspire a lot and you feel anxious. Sometimes you are even sick. These symptoms disappear as soon as you have a drink of alcohol.

You are in hospital because you vomited blood at home. You are very concerned about your declining physical health. You think it may be related to your alcohol consumption.

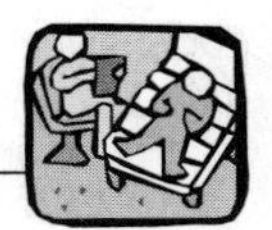

Construct

This OSCE assesses the candidate's ability to elicit the complications of alcohol misuse. The candidate should demonstrate a non-judgemental approach and handle the situation with sensitivity.

Examiner's marking sheet

	Excellent	Good	Satisfactory	Fail	Poor
Communication skills					
Assessment of physical complications					
Assessment of psychological complications					
Assessment of social complications					
Overall mark					

Communication skills

The development of alcohol dependency is nearly always accompanied by complications, which may be physical, psychological and/or social in nature. Such problems can be distressing for the patient to recall, so it is important to take a non-judgemental approach and be empathetic – that is, to understand and share the feelings of the patient. For example:

> 'That period in your life, when you had so many pressures at work, seems to have been very difficult for you.'

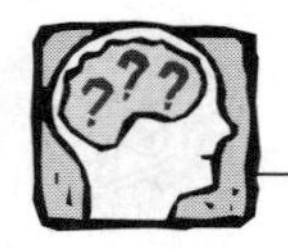

'I can appreciate that when your wife left you, you must have been distressed. How did you cope at the time?'

Assessment of physical complications

Patients find it relatively easy to talk about 'medical' problems, which they normally take to mean physical symptoms. Open questions about health problems and visits to the patient's GP or to hospitals will usually result in a lot of information, although the patient may not associate all of their symptoms with alcohol consumption.

Physical complications may include any of the following:

- cardiovascular complications – hypertension, cardiomegaly
- respiratory complications – tuberculosis (through vagrancy)
- gastrointestinal complications – oesophageal varices, oesophageal carcinoma, gastritis, peptic ulceration, liver problems (fatty degeneration, alcoholic hepatitis, cirrhosis, hepatoma), pancreatitis
- neurological complications – head injury, peripheral neuropathy, epilepsy, cerebellar degeneration
- miscellaneous – rhinophyma, gout, vitamin deficiencies.

Assessment of psychological complications

Patients remember psychological problems because they can be very distressing, but they may not volunteer them as complications of alcohol misuse. Do not accept basic answers, but explore each of the complications to assess the severity.

Psychological complications may include any of the following:

- acute intoxication
- pathological intoxication – this occurs very soon after drinking amounts of alcohol that are insufficient to cause intoxication in most people, and it may lead to verbally aggressive or physically violent behaviour that is not typical of the person when sober
- memory blackouts – these are discrete episodes of memory loss associated with severe intoxication; they are more common in binge drinkers
- withdrawal symptoms – these occur in the hours after drinking has stopped, and include tremor of the hands, sweating, nausea,

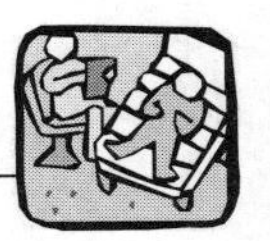

retching, vomiting, tachycardia, hypertension, psychomotor agitation, headache, insomnia, malaise or weakness, transient hallucinations or illusions, and convulsions

- delirium tremens ('the DTs') – this is a toxic confusional state that occurs 2 to 3 days after drinking has stopped
- Wernicke's encephalopathy – this is due to a deficiency of thiamine in the diet, and is characterised by a triad of acute mental confusion, ataxia and ophthalmoplegia
- Korsakoff's psychosis
- alcoholic dementia.

Assessment of social complications

Question the patient on various aspects of his lifestyle in turn. Be alert for evasive answers that may hide serious issues.

Social complications may include accidents, family and relationship problems – violence towards others, psychosexual difficulties. Schooling is also a problem with truancy and drinking in gangs. Employment problems include poor time-keeping, poor attendance, poor performance, days off work, dismissals and periods of unemployment.

There are also social problems such as housing issues, homelessness and vagrancy. Criminal problems include drink-related behaviour, crime to fund expenditure on alcohol, drink-driving offences, sexual assaults and violence.

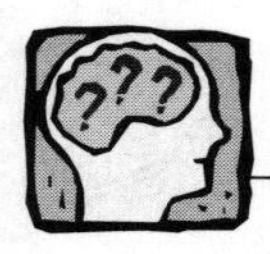

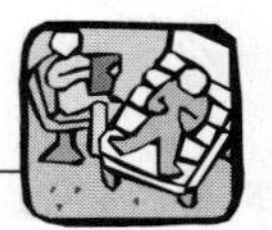

OSCE 22

Instructions for candidate

A confused man has been brought to casualty by the police. He was found near the town hall in a dishevelled state.

Perform a Mini Mental State Examination on this patient. Inform the examiner of the final score and discuss the implications of the score.

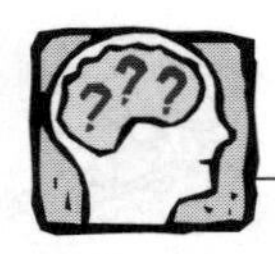

Instructions for actor

You are a 65-year-old man. In recent months you have been having increasing difficulty with your memory, so that your short-term memory is now poor. Earlier this morning you went to a shop to buy bread. You became disorientated and started to panic. You forgot how to get back to your house, but fortunately a police officer offered assistance.

You are co-operative and polite. If you are asked questions about the time, date and day of the week, you give the wrong answers. If you are asked about your present location, you also give the wrong answer, telling the doctor that you are in the police station. If you are asked to memorise anything, you can recall everything immediately, but if you are asked again after a few minutes, you can only recall one of the items. You answer all other questions normally.

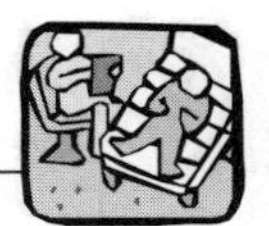

Construct

This OSCE assesses the candidate's ability to give clear instructions to a confused patient and to carry out a competent examination.

Examiner's marking sheet

	Excellent	Good	Satisfactory	Fail	Poor
Communication skills					
Asking the correct Mini Mental State Examination questions					
Marking the answers correctly and giving the correct final score					
Overall mark					

Communication skills

Interviewing a confused patient can be difficult if you do not spend a few minutes at the beginning introducing yourself and the purpose of your test. Establishing rapport and making the patient feel comfortable are important and will help you to gain the patient's informed consent to proceed with the examination. It is a good idea to indicate to the patient that some of the questions may seem rather basic and others more difficult, but that they are all part of a standard test. Be careful not to rush the patient. Remember to offer reassurance if he appears to be struggling with the answers, but do not give any prompts or cues. Make a note of any hearing impairment which may make it difficult to obtain a reliable score.

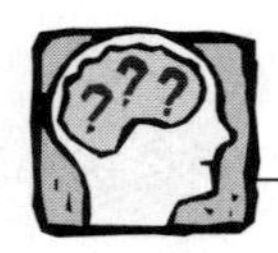

Asking the correct Mini Mental State Examination questions

Orientation in time (maximum score = 5)

Ask the patient to tell you the date. Probe if necessary. Award one mark for each of the following: Year, season, month, date, day.

Orientation in place (maximum score = 5)

Award one mark for each of the following: Country, county, city/town, building, floor.

Registration (maximum score = 3)

Inform the patient that you would like to test his memory by asking him to repeat three words which you are going to say. Give the patient three unrelated words (eg 'ball, car, table'), and ask him to repeat the words back to you. If he fails to do this, repeat the process until he has learned all three words. Award one mark for each word repeated during the first attempt. If the patient fails to repeat all three words, the recall test below will be meaningless.

Attention (maximum score = 5)

Ask the patient whether he can spell the word 'world'. If he can, ask him to spell the word backwards. Award one mark for each letter spoken in the correct reverse order.

Alternatively, you may ask the patient to subtract 7 from 100 repeatedly, telling you each answer as he does so. Award one mark for each correct answer, up to a maximum of five marks in five answers.

Recall (maximum score = 3)

Ask the patient to recall the three words you asked him to remember earlier. Award one mark for each correctly recalled word.

Naming (maximum score = 2)

Ask the patient to name two objects to which you point, eg a wrist-watch and a pen. Award one mark for each correct answer.

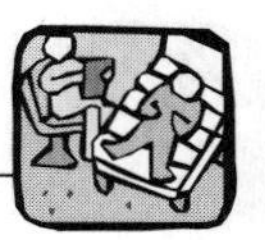

Repetition (maximum score = 1)

Ask the patient to repeat the following sentence: 'no ifs, ands or buts.' Award one mark if he is successful on the first attempt.

Three-stage command (maximum score = 3)

Give the patient the following instruction: 'Take this sheet of paper from me in your left hand, fold it in half and place it on the floor.' Hold a sheet of paper for the patient to take from you. Award one mark for each correct action.

Reading (maximum score = 1)

On a sheet of paper write the phrase 'CLOSE YOUR EYES' in large print. Ask the patient to read the phrase and to do what it says. Award one mark if he closes his eyes.

Writing (maximum score = 1)

Ask the patient to write a sentence on a sheet of paper. Award one mark if the sentence makes sense and includes a noun and a verb, even if there are spelling and/or grammatical errors.

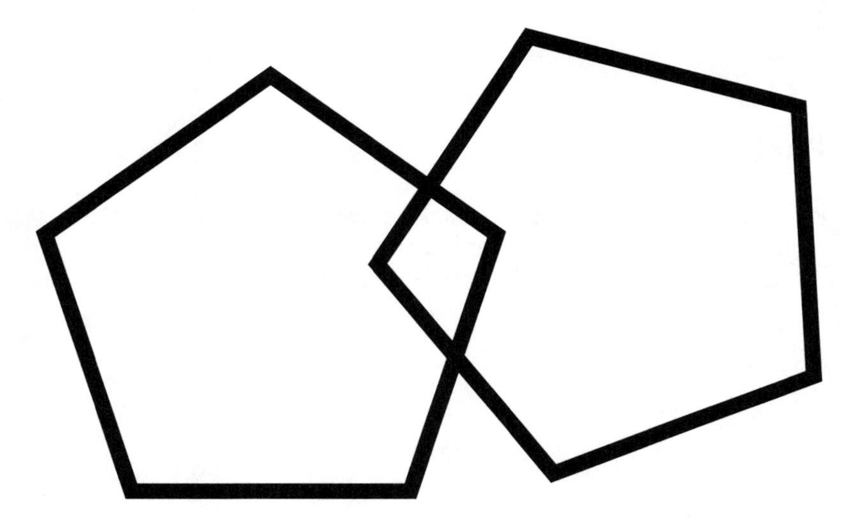

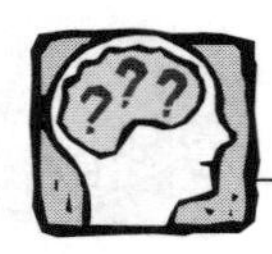

Copying (maximum score = 1)

On a sheet of paper draw two intersecting pentagons. Ask the patient to copy the diagram. Award one mark if all ten angles are drawn, with two angles intersecting to form a four-sided shape. Ignore shaky lines or rotation of the figure.

Marking the answers correctly and giving the correct final score

Final score

The maximum possible score is 30. Remember to give the examiner the final score.

The degree of cognitive impairment can be assessed on the basis of the final score as follows:

- score of 24 to 30 – within normal limits
- score of 18 to 23 – mild to moderate cognitive impairment
- score of 0 to 17 – severe cognitive impairment.

You should also mention your assessment of the level of consciousness of the patient, which will be somewhere on a continuum from coma to fully alert. Delirium may result in a low score.

Further reading

Folstein, M.F., Folstein, S.E. and McHugh, P.R. 1975. Mini-Mental State: a practical method for grading the state of patients for the clinician. *Journal of Psychiatric Research,* 12, 189–198.

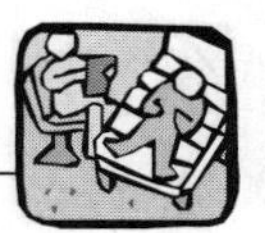

OSCE 23

Instructions for candidate

You are interviewing a patient in the outpatient clinic who has recently been diagnosed with Alzheimer's disease. She mentions that she is putting her finances in order. Assess the patient's ability to make a will (testamentary capacity).

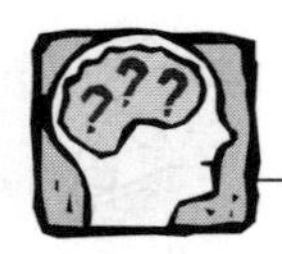

Instructions for actor

You are a 75-year-old widow. You live alone in a house you purchased 10 years ago for £100,000. You have three sons, all of whom are married and have children. You see two of your sons frequently. They live locally with their families. Your youngest son is the black sheep of the family. He was imprisoned in 1992 for credit card fraud, and you have very little contact with him.

During the last few months you have become increasingly forgetful. You were not worried about this until your eldest son expressed his concerns. You then went to see your family doctor, who referred you to a psychiatrist at the local hospital. After a series of tests, this doctor diagnosed the early stages of Alzheimer's disease. You have been told that the disease is progressive, and that at the moment it can be managed at home. However, this might not always be the case.

You have decided to put your finances in order. You wish to make a will with the following arrangements:

- You wish the house, which you erroneously think is still valued at £100,000, to go to your two eldest sons.
- Of the savings you have left, you want to give £10,000 to each of your two eldest sons.
- You wish to give nothing to your youngest son.
- You wish to give £1000 to each of your grandchildren.
- You wish to give £5000 to the plumber who fixed your blocked toilet last week.

You are confused about the correct time and you keep on forgetting who you are talking to – you repeatedly ask the doctor who he is and why he is in your house. You answer questions about your family correctly and you know how you wish your assets to be distributed after your death. You cannot explain why you want to give money to the plumber and you keep changing your mind about how much to give him.

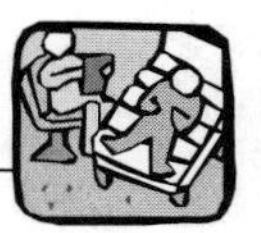

Construct

This OSCE assesses the candidate's ability to patiently assess testamentary capacity in a woman suffering from Alzheimer's disease.

Examiner's marking sheet

	Excellent	Good	Satisfactory	Fail	Poor
Communication skills					
Establishing the property of the patient					
Evaluating the proposed distribution of the property					
Summarising the clinical findings					
Overall mark					

Communication skills

Making a will is a sensitive issue for most people, as it is an acknowledgement that, try as one might, one cannot avoid death. For a person with dementia, it may also mark the realisation that the progressive nature of the disease means that plans for the future will have to be made now.

As well as establishing rapport, you need to establish early in the interview that this patient understands the nature and implications of making a will.

Establishing the property of the patient

Testamentary capacity has to be determined with regard to a particular will. You will need to establish the extent and value of the

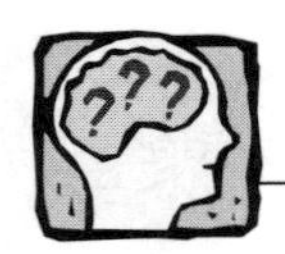

patient's property because the more complex the disposition, the greater the mental capacity necessary. An initial step may be to ask an open question. For example:

> 'Can you talk to me about what you own or what you are planning to give away in your will?'

It is important to check the factual correctness of each item that the patient lists. This patient has Alzheimer's disease, so she may not accurately recall details about her property.

Evaluating the proposed distribution of the property

You should then ask the patient whether she knows the individuals who are the objects of her will. She should appreciate which individuals may reasonably expect to benefit, and the manner of distribution of her property between them. Anything that sounds unusual must be investigated further. In the psychiatric assessment any abnormality of the mind that impairs the decision-making process must be noted. It does not matter if the person making the will does not act wisely or prudently. In this example, you need to probe the patient's reasons for giving money to the plumber.

Summarising the clinical findings

A decision as to whether a person has testamentary capacity is made on the balance of probabilities. You should therefore address the question 'Is it more probable than not that this patient lacks or has testamentary capacity?'. The standard of proof is not 'beyond reasonable doubt.' Note that the presence of mental illness or detention under the Mental Health Act 1983 does not mean that the person lacks testamentary capacity.

You may need to review the patient's medical notes and talk to the solicitor and third parties to obtain background information.

Further reading

British Geriatrics Society Guidelines on Testamentary Capacity; www.bgs.org.uk

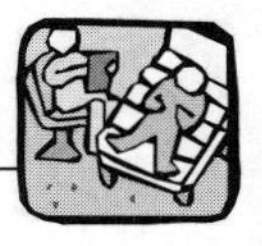

British Geriatrics Society Compendium Document, Document G3 (1997); www.bgs.org.uk

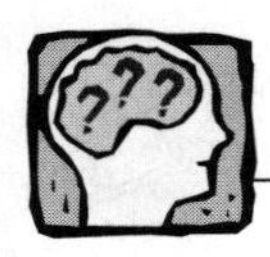

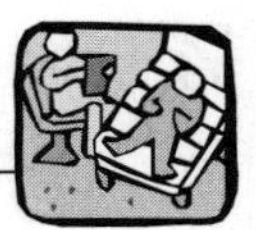

OSCE 24

Instructions for candidate

A 20-year-old student has come to see you in the outpatient clinic. For as long as she can remember she has been a tidy person. However, for the last two years cleanliness has dominated her life. Take a history of obsessions and compulsions from this patient.

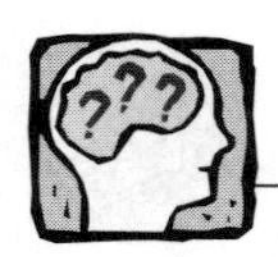

Instructions for actor

You are a 20-year-old student. You recently asked your GP for help because you cannot stop washing your hands. Every day you wash them at least 20 times, sometimes spending up to 20 minutes at the basin. You keep thinking that your hands are full of germs. Although you know that in fact they are clean and you try to resist these thoughts, you cannot do so. You think that you are going crazy.

You remember being tidy even as a child. Your bedroom used to be very neat, with everything laid out in an orderly fashion. When you started university, you shared a flat with friends. You were appalled by their attitude to hygiene in the kitchen and bathroom, and you ended up doing most of the cleaning yourself. You became increasingly concerned about contaminating your hands, and took to washing them regularly using antibacterial soap.

You also spend a lot of time in the shower each morning, much to the annoyance of your flatmates. You have a ritual in which you have to wash your body in a certain way. If at any point this ritual is interrupted, you have to start again. One day last week you spent an hour in the shower.

You are always the last to leave the flat because you keep thinking that you have not switched off the hairdryer, turned off the light switches or locked the door properly. You repeatedly check these items and sometimes you even return from lectures to check them again.

You are co-operative during the interview, and you answer all of the questions as best you can.

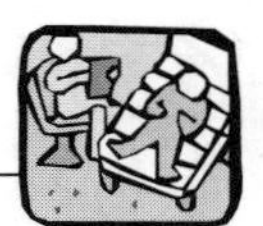

Construct

This OSCE assesses the candidate's ability to elicit the symptoms of obsessive-compulsive disorder. The candidate should be able to assess the impact of these symptoms on the patient's life.

Examiner's marking sheet

	Excellent	Good	Satisfactory	Fail	Poor
Communication skills					
Eliciting the symptoms of obsessive-compulsive disorder					
Assessing the impact of these symptoms on daily life					
Overall mark					

Communication skills

You should introduce yourself to the patient and gather information using a combination of open and closed questions. Some patients with obsessive-compulsive disorder see no problem with their symptoms, while others are distressed by them. It is important to demonstrate empathy during your questioning, and to address any concerns that the patient may have.

Eliciting the symptoms of obsessive-compulsive disorder

Obsessional thoughts are ideas, images or impulses that enter the patient's mind repeatedly. Compulsive acts or rituals are behaviours

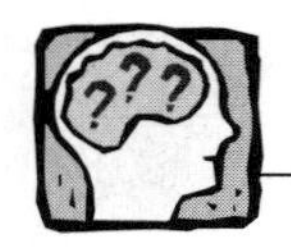

that are repeated again and again. The symptoms typically involve cleaning and checking. It is important to elicit detailed information about each symptom, so that you can determine whether the patient is describing true obsessions and compulsions.

'Can you describe to me what has been happening to you?'

'Tell me about the thoughts you have been having.'

For a diagnosis of obsessive-compulsive disorder, either the obsessions or the compulsions, or both, must have been present on most days for a period of at least two weeks.

'How often do you have these thoughts? When did they start?'

Obsessions and compulsions share the following features, which must all be present:

- They are acknowledged as originating in the mind of the patient.

  'Where do your thoughts come from?'

- They are repetitive and unpleasant.

  'What is it like to have these thoughts?'

- The patient tries unsuccessfully to resist them.

  'Do you try anything to stop or resist these thoughts?'

- At least one obsession or compulsion is acknowledged as being excessive or unreasonable.

  'Does it make sense to you to have these thoughts or to carry out these behaviours?'

- Experiencing the obsessive thoughts or carrying out the compulsive act is not in itself pleasurable.

If you have time, you should also demonstrate that the obsessions and compulsions are not the result of other mental disorders, such as schizophrenia, mood disorders or other anxiety disorders.

Assessing the impact of these symptoms on daily life

One way of assessing the impact of the symptoms is to ask the patient to talk you through a typical day. Gather information on the

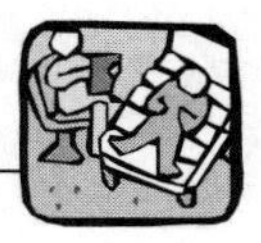

frequency and duration of symptoms and the patient's coping strategies. Ask her whether her symptoms prevent her from taking part in any other activities. Finally, enquire about the attitudes of other people and also about the psychological impact of having the disorder.

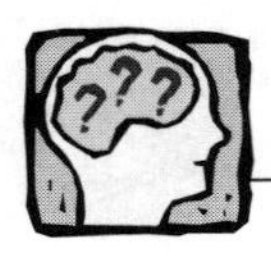

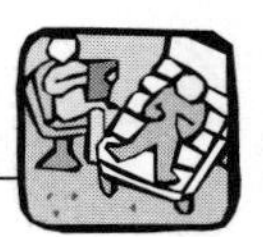

OSCE 25

Instructions for candidate

You have been asked to see a 23-year-old woman in casualty. She was brought to the hospital by ambulance earlier this evening after she took an overdose. She has accepted treatment for the paracetamol overdose, but the casualty officer remains concerned about her mental health. Assess this act of deliberate self-harm, and discuss the management options with the patient.

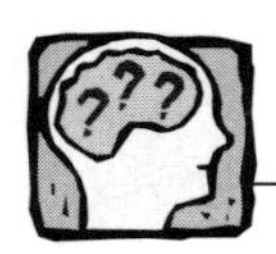

Instructions for actor

You are a 23-year-old woman. You are in the casualty unit of your local hospital waiting to see a psychiatrist.

You have been depressed for three years. You are taking an antidepressant called citalopram which normally controls your mood. Three months ago you were made redundant and your mood deteriorated. You feel worst first thing in the morning, and you find it difficult to motivate yourself. You have been sleeping poorly and neglecting yourself by not eating and not washing regularly. You have been experiencing feelings of hopelessness and helplessness, and you feel guilty about being a burden on your boyfriend. You have had thoughts of harming yourself, and yesterday you purchased paracetamol tablets from four different pharmacies. You thought that life was no longer worth living and that everyone would be happier when you were gone.

Early this evening, after your boyfriend had left the house to watch a football game, you took 64 paracetamol tablets. You then went to bed. You left a suicide note that you had prepared earlier on the bedside table. You thought that you would fall asleep and never wake up again.

You were woken up by your boyfriend. He was shaking you, asking you if you had taken tablets. He had found the empty boxes of tablets in the kitchen and had become suspicious. You told him that you had taken the tablets. He phoned for an ambulance and you were brought to casualty.

You are distressed, and you are shocked and embarrassed by your actions. You answer the doctor's questions but you speak slowly and quietly. You sit with your head in your hands and you look sad. You try to convince the doctor that it is now safe for you to go home with your boyfriend. You no longer feel suicidal, but you are not sure how you will feel if you return home.

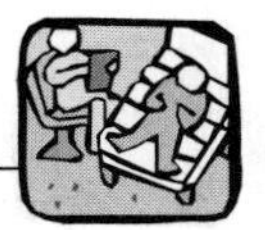

Construct

This OSCE tests the candidate's ability to assess the risks associated with an act of deliberate self-harm and to formulate a management plan based on those risks.

Examiner's marking sheet

	Excellent	Good	Satisfactory	Fail	Poor
Communication skills					
Assessment of the severity of the act of deliberate self-harm					
Assessment of the past psychiatric history and the aetiology of the present episode					
Formulation of an appropriate management plan					
Overall mark					

Communication skills

The patient has been through an extremely distressing experience, and you should acknowledge this. Use open questions to determine the events that led up to the incident and then closed questions to fill in the gaps. It is important to adopt a non-judgemental approach and be empathetic. Try to understand what has happened to make this woman consider taking her own life.

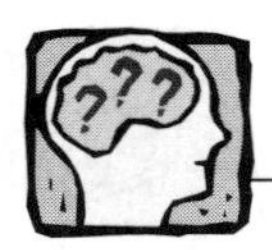

Assessment of the severity of the act of deliberate self-harm

Circumstances that suggest a high level of suicidal intent include the following:

- planning in advance
- precautions to avoid discovery
- carrying out the act while alone
- making no attempt to obtain help afterwards
- using a dangerous or violent method
- 'final acts' (eg suicide note, making a will, giving away possessions).

The following demographic features also increase the risk, and you should ask about these if they are not obvious and the patient does not volunteer the information:

- male sex
- older age group (> 40 years)
- a history of previous attempts or a family history of suicide
- social isolation
- unemployment
- one or more causes of stress that cannot be resolved
- a lack of plans for the future, or a feeling of hopelessness
- physical illness (especially chronic painful illness, epilepsy or cancer)
- psychiatric illness.

Assessment of the past psychiatric history and the aetiology of the present episode

Around 90% of patients who commit suicide have a psychiatric disorder. Around 50% have depression, 25% have alcohol problems, 5% have schizophrenia and 20% have other disorders, including personality disorders, chronic neuroses and substance abuse disorders. Among psychiatric inpatients the suicide rate is 50 times higher than that in the general population.

It is therefore important to ask about previous mental health problems. Enquire about diagnoses, investigations, treatments and

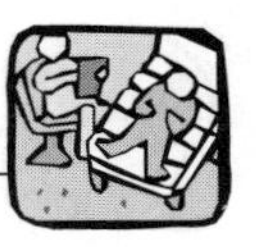

outcomes. Detention under the Mental Health Act 1983 signifies more severe difficulties, particularly under the treatment orders.

You must ask the patient about her motive for taking the overdose. Even a very small overdose is dangerous if the patient believed that it would kill her.

Motives for attempting suicide include the following:

- the wish to die
- a cry for help, to try to change an intolerable situation
- an attempt to influence other people
- an attempt to escape from emotional distress
- an expression of anger directed at another person or at oneself
- a test of the benevolence of 'fate' ('if I survive this, it was meant to be').

Formulation of an appropriate management plan

You need to consider psychiatric, psychological and social interventions that will reduce the risk of further self-harm. However, the most pressing issues are where the patient is to be treated and how urgently they need to be treated.

You should summarise the clinical findings to the patient, and ideally you should then have a discussion with her and come to an agreement about the best way forward. Do not dismiss any of her suggestions without carefully giving your reasons for doing so. You should also explain the advantages and disadvantages of each management option.

> 'It's been a difficult evening for you. What do you wish to happen now?'

If the patient insists on only one plan, such as going home, ask her how she can be helped if she does go home. For example, the community mental health team may be able to offer additional support.

> 'You say you want to go home. What kind of help do you think you would benefit from at home?'
>
> 'People often feel better when they're in casualty, but when they return home the same problems resurface. How will you cope with

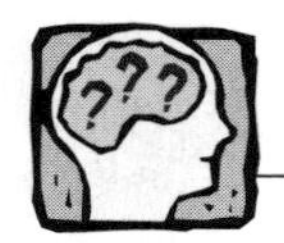

that? What has changed so that you are not at the same level of risk?'

Gently probe other possibilities, such as hospital admission.

'Are there any other options you might consider, such as staying in hospital?'

If the patient refuses to be admitted voluntarily to hospital and you consider that she needs to be hospitalised, you will have to detain her under the Mental Health Act. You should explain what this means, pausing often to make sure that the patient understands you.

'I am concerned about you. I think that you are unwell and at risk. Because of what you have told me, my recommendation is that you stay in hospital so that we can help you further.

Normally patients are admitted voluntarily to hospital, but sometimes the judgement of a patient can be affected, so that his or her decision-making capabilities are impaired. In such circumstances we need to ensure the safety, assessment and treatment of these patients. We use the Mental Health Act 1983 to detain these patients in the interests of their own health or safety or with a view to the protection of others.

'However, I cannot do this by myself. I will talk to another doctor and an Approved Social Worker (ASW) who will also want to speak with you. If we all agree that you need to be in hospital, then the ASW can make the application for admission to hospital under the Act.

'If you think that you are being unfairly detained in hospital, you will be able to appeal to the hospital managers and/or the Mental Health Review Tribunal, which is an independent panel that safeguards the interests of patients.'

You should offer the patient a source of further information, such as a patient information leaflet that explains her rights.

You may go on to explain what treatments can be offered – for example, reviewing her antidepressant treatment, starting an intervention such as cognitive behavioural therapy, and rehabilitating her so that she can return to work.

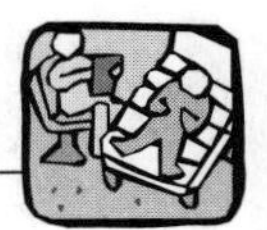

OSCE 26

Instructions for candidate

A man is brought to casualty who says that he is hearing voices – 'they're going to get me!' Elicit the first-rank symptoms of schizophrenia.

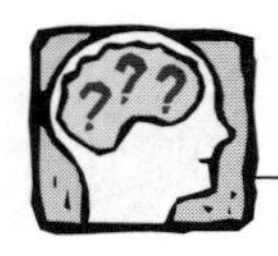

Instructions for actor

You are a 25-year-old man who has been brought into the Accident and Emergency department by the police. You believe that you have special powers as a result of a chip that has been installed in your brain by MI5.

You feel that your thoughts are not your own, some of the thoughts in your head having been placed there by MI5, so that they can now read your mind. You can hear agents from MI5 discussing your importance and your mission among themselves.

You have been admitted to hospital once before under a section of the Mental Health Act. You were discharged on medication, but you do not believe that you have a mental illness. At present you are angry that you have been brought to the Accident and Emergency department by the police against your will.

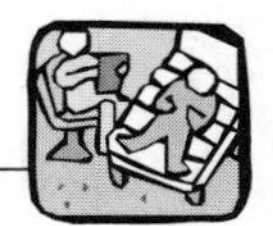

Construct

This OSCE assesses the candidate's ability to demonstrate an adequate knowledge of the first-rank symptoms of schizophrenia. They should empathise with the patient and at the same time be able to control the interview process. In addition, they should be able to take a good history that will enable them to establish a diagnosis of schizophrenia.

Examiner's marking sheet

	Excellent	Good	Satisfactory	Fail	Poor
Communication skills					
Demonstration of abnormalities in thought					
Demonstration of first-rank auditory hallucinations					
Demonstration of passivity phenomenon					
Demonstration of delusional perceptions					
Overall mark					

Communication skills

General principles of establishing good rapport and communication with the patient are essential. The actor may have been instructed

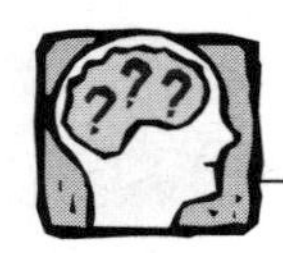

to be guarded and hostile, so be aware of this and never lose your temper or display irritable or temperamental behaviour towards the patient.

Diagnosis of schizophrenia

For a diagnosis of schizophrenia to be made, one of the first-rank symptoms must be present for at least **one month**. First-rank symptoms include the following:

- thought insertion, withdrawal and broadcasting
- auditory hallucinations (eg running commentary, thought echo and third-person auditory hallucinations)
- delusional perceptions
- passivity phenomenon.

It is important to establish that you can take a good history without resorting to the use of jargon (a common trap when eliciting psychopathology at an OSCE station).

Remember always to explain to the patient exactly what you mean, using examples, so that they understand clearly what you are asking. Thus you should establish first-rank symptoms in layman terms.

Demonstration of abnormalities in thought

You need to show the examiner that you are able to ask the right questions to demonstrate the abnormalities in thought which are of first-rank importance. Before you start asking more direct questions, a good opening question would be as follows:

> 'Do you feel that your thoughts are muddled or being interfered with?'

This general question can be followed by more specific questions about thought broadcasting, thought insertion and thought withdrawal.

Thought broadcasting
This can be demonstrated by asking the following question.

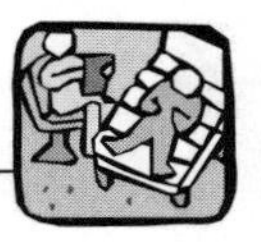

'Have you ever felt that your thoughts were being beamed or broadcast so that other people can hear them?'

Thought insertion
This symptom can be elicited by asking the following questions:

'Do you think that sometimes maybe your thoughts are not your own?'

'Do you feel that thoughts can be put into your mind? Do you think these thoughts are being put there by some outside force or person?'

Thought withdrawal
This can usually be demonstrated by asking:

'Do you ever feel that your mind goes blank?'

Follow on by asking:

'Do you ever feel that your mind goes empty or that it has been drained of thoughts?'

Alternatively, you could ask:

'Have you ever felt that your thoughts were taken away by some outside force or person?'

Demonstration of first-rank auditory hallucinations

Remember that you have been asked to demonstrate the first-rank symptoms, so it is crucial that you do this before clarifying any other symptoms.

Before you ask more direct questions about specific types of auditory hallucinations, start with an open question to establish that the patient experiences auditory hallucinations:

'Sometimes can you hear voices talking to you when there is no one else in the room?'

Once you have established that the patient is experiencing auditory hallucinations, follow up with more direct questioning to establish specific types of auditory hallucinations which are of first rank.

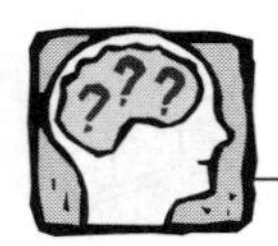

Running commentary
You can test this by asking the following questions:

> 'Do your voices ever talk or comment on what you do?'

You could elaborate and give an example to clarify to the patient exactly what you mean. Another useful approach is to ask for the actual content:

> 'What do they say?'

On the basis of the patient's answer you can then decipher the nature of the hallucination.

Third-person auditory hallucinations
These can be elicited by asking:

> 'Do your voices talk amongst themselves and do they talk about you?'

Again give an example to clarify your meaning, and ask for the actual content of what was said.

Thought echo
This symptom can usually be tested for by asking the following question:

> 'Can you sometimes hear your thoughts out aloud – as if they were a voice outside your head?'

Demonstration of passivity phenomenon

Here you have to demonstrate the subjective feeling that the patient has about his feelings, thoughts and actions being controlled by an external agent or force. This needs to be done by asking the following questions:

> 'Have you ever felt that you were being controlled by some outside force?'

> 'Do you feel that an outside force or person is controlling you?'

If the answer is yes, clarify by asking whether they control the patient's thoughts, movements or feelings.

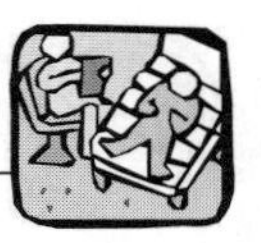

Another good tactic is to give an example such as the following:

'Do you feel like a puppet on a string or a robot being controlled by a remote?'

Demonstration of delusional perceptions

This is generally one of the most difficult first-rank symptoms to demonstrate. By definition a delusional perception has to be 'de novo' and not have arisen from previous states. To demonstrate a delusional perception you need to screen for the presence of other types of delusions, such as delusions of grandiosity or persecution. After the patient has volunteered a delusion, you then need to establish whether it has arisen suddenly, 'out of the blue'.

This can be achieved by asking more about the actual content of the delusion and doing some reality testing.

In the OSCE, you need to demonstrate that you are systematic and thorough, and in the 7-minute time-frame keep to the sequence described above.

It is sometimes necessary to clarify what you mean by rephrasing the above questions. Practice makes perfect, so make sure that you have a set of stock questions which you can reel out with ease and confidence.

Further reading

Andreasen, N.C. and Black D.W. 2001. *Introductory textbook of psychiatry*, third edn. American Psychiatric Publishing Inc., pp59–67.

Carlat, J.D. 1999. *The psychiatric interview*. Lippincott Williams and Wilkins, pp183–201.

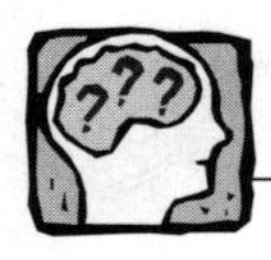

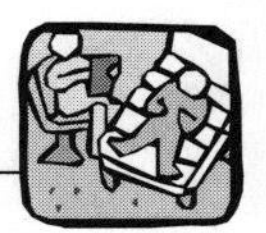

OSCE 27

Instructions for candidate

Examine this patient who has recently been started on an antipsychotic and is complaining of stiffness in his neck and jaw. Give a running commentary as you examine the patient.

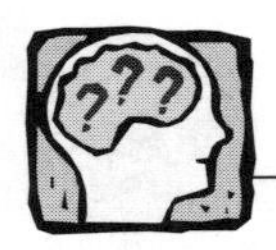

Construct

The candidate should be able to show that they have a good understanding of extrapyramidal side-effects and are able to demonstrate them by examining the patient in a systematic manner.

Usually the simulated patient will be normal and will not show any signs or symptoms.

Examiner's marking sheet

	Excellent	Good	Satisfactory	Fail	Poor
Communication skills					
Examination for tremors					
Examination for rigidity					
Examination for hypokinesia					
Examination of gait					
Overall mark					

Communication skills

Introduce yourself to the patient and explain to them what you are about to do. General principles of empathy and good communication are essential.

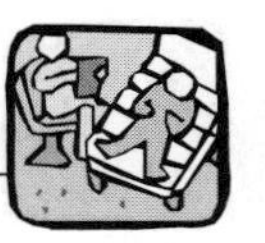

Examination for tremors, rigidity, hypokinesia and gait

This needs to be done in an orderly and systematic manner.

1 Explain to the patient what you are going to do.

2 Observe the patient at rest, noting any abnormal involuntary movements of the limbs or trunk.

3 Ask the patient if he has anything in his mouth, such as chewing-gum, and if so to remove it. Now ask him whether he has noticed any abnormal movements, and if so, to what extent they affect him.

4 Ask the patient to sit in a chair, first with his hands on his knees and then with the hands hanging unsupported. Note any abnormal movements in the limbs or trunk.

5 Ask the patient to open his mouth, and examine his tongue for any resting tremors. Then ask him to protrude his tongue, and note any abnormalities in movement (both should be done twice).

6 Ask the patient to tap his thumb with each finger as rapidly as possible. Observe him carefully for any abnormal movements as he is performing the task. It is important to make sure that the patient understands what you are asking him to do (give a demonstration of the thumb tapping and then ask him to repeat it).

7 Examine both the upper and lower limbs for tone, examining one limb at a time by passively flexing and extending the limb and feeling for the tone in the muscle groups.

8 Ask the patient to stand up, and again note any abnormal posturing or movements.

9 Ask the patient to extend both arms with the palms facing downward, and note any tremors. Observe all areas, not just the arms.

10 Now ask the patient to walk up and down the room twice, and note his gait. It is important to record comments about the arm-swing at this point.

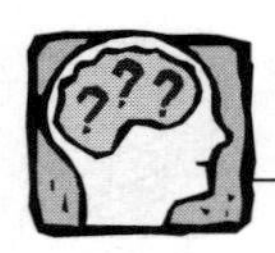

Avoiding common pitfalls

It is important to keep the patient at ease at all times. Seven minutes is ample time to complete the entire task. Be systematic and make sure that all areas of the examination are covered. If you are asked to give a running commentary, make sure that you speak loudly and clearly and that you make eye contact with the examiner.

Further reading

Owens, D.G.C. 1999. *A guide to the extrapyramidal side-effects of antipsychotic medication*. Cambridge, Cambridge University Press.

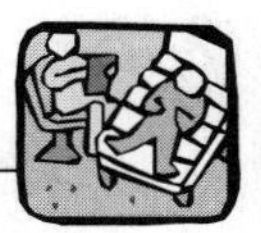

OSCE 28

Instructions for candidate

Mrs Green is a 34-year-old woman who has been diagnosed with depression. You are seeing her in the outpatient clinic and would like to start her on an antidepressant. Explain to the patient how antidepressants work and how she will benefit from them.

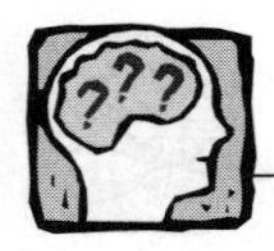

Instructions for actor

You are a 34-year-old woman who has just been diagnosed with depression. Your psychiatrist has suggested that you start taking an antidepressant. You have never been depressed in the past and this is your first episode of depression. You have concerns about the medication as you think it may be addictive, and you are not very sure how it will work and whether it will help you. You would also like to know how quickly antidepressants act and for how long you have to take them.

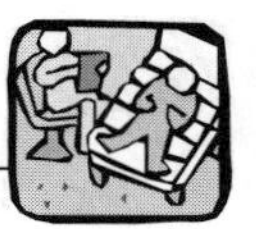

Construct

This OSCE assesses the candidate's ability to establish rapport and empathise with the patient. The candidate should also be able to communicate the mechanism of action and the principles of antidepressant treatment in a simple and succinct way.

Examiner's marking sheet

	Excellent	Good	Satisfactory	Fail	Poor
Communication skills					
Explanation of the mechanism of action of antidepressants					
Ability to answer the patient's questions					
Overall mark					

Communication skills

The key element that is being tested in this scenario is how well you communicate with the patient. It is essential to establish rapport with the patient, and to be able to communicate in a straightforward manner, without using jargon, when you are explaining the pathophysiology of depression and the mechanism of action of antidepressants.

A good approach would be to introduce yourself and summarise the patient's history.

You could then explain to the patient that she has been diagnosed with depression and that you have been asked to explain to her how antidepressants work.

The actor will have been instructed to ask some relevant questions about the treatment. It is important to remember that you are being marked on how well you are able to clarify any uncertainties or doubts that the patient might have about her treatment.

Explanation of the mechanism of action of antidepressants

You could explain this as follows:

> 'When a person is feeling low or depressed, certain chemicals in their brain called neurotransmitters are at low levels. Antidepressants work by bringing these levels back to normal. There are several different types of antidepressants, such as tricyclic antidepressants (TCAs) and selective serotonin reuptake inhibitors (SSRIs). In your case we would like to start an SSRI called paroxetine'.

The actress has been primed to ask a number of questions

For how long will I have to take antidepressants?

'Antidepressants take anywhere between two and six weeks to work, so it is essential that you persist with the medication without stopping. Once they start to work you will need to take them for at least another 6 to 8 months for them to be effective. Before you stop any medication or make any changes to it you will need to speak to your psychiatrist again'.

Are antidepressants addictive?

'Antidepressants are not addictive. However, as with all medication it is important to remember that you should not stop them suddenly. You should always take the advice of your doctor before you make any changes to your medication'.

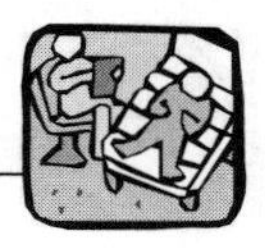

Do antidepressants have any side-effects?

The antidepressant that we would like to start you on is generally a very safe medication. However, in some people it can upset their tummy and cause nausea and diarrhoea. But this does not happen to everyone, and usually the symptoms improve after a couple of days. Also in some people it can make them slightly agitated initially, and to prevent this we tend to start patients on a small dose and then gradually build it up'.

I have heard that antidepressants can make one suicidal. Is this true?

'Antidepressants are an effective form of treatment for depression and are very unlikely to make people suicidal. Certain antidepressants can make some people feel anxious in the first couple of days of treatment. However, to prevent this happening we generally start the treatment at a small dose and then gradually build it up'.

Can I drive while taking my medication?

'According to the DVLA guidelines, anxiety or depression that is not associated with significant memory or concentration problems, agitation, behavioural disturbance or suicidal ideation does not need to be notified to the DVLA'.

Therefore the advice given in the OSCE scenario will be dependent on these factors. All patients who are currently suicidal or have severe forms of depression will have to notify the DVLA of their condition and will have to cease driving until the outcome of the medical enquiry is known.

We were thinking of having another baby soon. Is the drug safe for the baby?

'Antidepressants have been used widely throughout pregnancy without any problems to the mother or the baby. If you were planning to become pregnant, we would first review how you were doing. If it was decided that you still require an antidepressant, you would be treated with one of the tricyclic antidepressants, for which there is the most evidence to show that they are safe in pregnancy'.

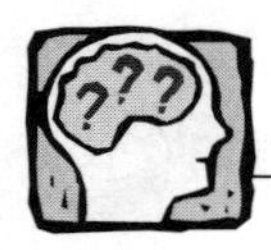

Further reading

Cohen, L.S. and Rosenbaum, J.F. 1998. Psychotropic drug use during pregnancy: weighing the risks. *Journal of Clinical Psychiatry*, 59 (Supplement 2), 18–28.

DVLA. *Psychiatric conditions and driving at a glance*; www.dvla.gov.uk/at_a_glance/ch4_psychiatric.htm.

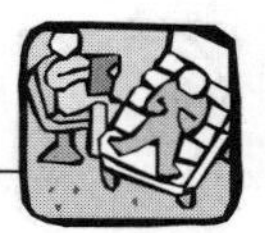

OSCE 29

Instructions for candidate

Explain to this 28-year-old woman who is currently being treated for depression the benefits of sleep hygiene and how she can improve her sleep pattern.

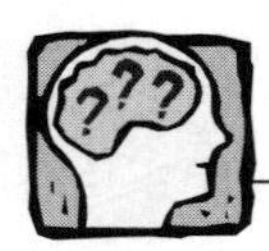

Instructions for actor

You are a 28-year-old woman who is currently on an antidepressant. For the past eight weeks while you have been taking the medication your mood seems to have improved. However, your sleeping is still a problem (and this has been the case for the last year or so). At present you have difficulty in falling asleep and you keep waking up through the night.

The doctor has been asked to give you some advice on how you can improve your sleep pattern. They will be asking you about your lifestyle and will want to know things like how much coffee or tea you drink, whether you smoke, the amount of alcohol you drink, and what you tend to do in the evenings before going to bed.

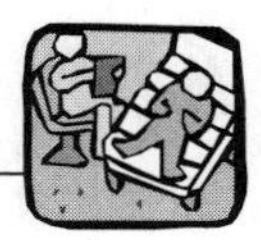

Construct

The candidate should be able to demonstrate that they are able to take a good history to establish certain factors that may be impacting on this patient's sleep pattern. They should give simple and sound advice to the patient, and should be able to answer any questions that the patient might have.

Examiner's marking sheet

	Excellent	Good	Satisfactory	Fail	Poor
Communication skills					
Thorough relevant history					
Advice on improving sleep hygiene					
Ability to answer the patient's questions					
Overall mark					

Communication skills

The majority of marks will be given for communication skills. Some of the main aspects that will be assessed include how well you establish rapport, whether you take a thorough relevant history, and your ability to explain to the patient the key factors related to sleep hygiene.

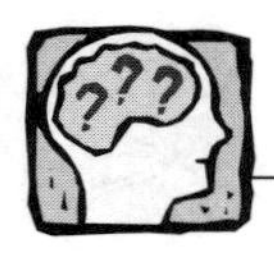

Thorough relevant history

When you have introduced yourself and briefly explained your role and the purpose of your interview, you should take a detailed relevant history. This will enable you to identify potential areas that can be modified by the patient so that she can improve her sleep pattern.

When establishing the relevant factors that might be affecting the patient's sleep pattern, the crucial areas that need to be covered include the following:

- current psychiatric history
- medical history
- current medication – ask about both prescribed and over-the-counter medication
- drug and alcohol history
- lifestyle and habits
- evening and bedtime activities.

It is important that you take a relevant history to demonstrate to the examiner that you are not just reeling off a list of facts to the patient, but are devising a management plan based on the problems posed by the patient's history.

Advice on improving sleep hygiene

Sleep is essential for good health, and the advice that you give to the patient should highlight this fact. The amount of sleep that an adult needs varies from one individual to another. For the average adult it is usually between 6 and 8 hours of sleep. To determine how much sleep you need in a night, make a note of how you feel the next morning. If you feel rested and alert, that is probably the amount of sleep you need. Advice on improving sleep hygiene should be given to the patient in plain and simple language, and should include the following elements:

- Avoid alcohol or nicotine just before bedtime.
- Consume less caffeine or caffeinated drinks in the evening. Also avoid drinking large amounts of fluids just before going to bed.
- Avoid doing vigorous exercise in the evening, as this will make you more aroused and less likely to fall asleep.

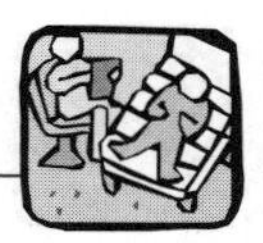

- Avoid heavy meals just before bedtime.
- Keep the bedroom free of clutter and work. It should be used for sleep and intimacy only. Make sure that there are minimal distractions, and do not watch television in bed.
- Develop a regular waking time, and avoid taking naps during the day.
- Try to do something relaxing just before bedtime (eg a hot shower or a soak in the bath).

The actor has been primed to ask a number of questions

The actor may be instructed to ask for sleeping tablets to help her with her sleep problems. Your advice should be that sleeping tablets are only used for short periods in patients who are acutely distressed, and are not effective long-term solutions as they make people dependent on them so they will keep requiring higher doses.

Further reading

Royal College of Psychiatrists. *Sleeping Well*, patient leaflet; www.rcpsych.ac.uk/info/help/sleep/index.htm

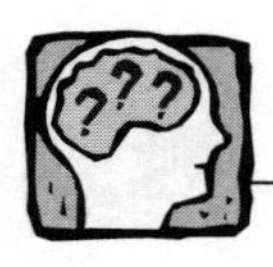

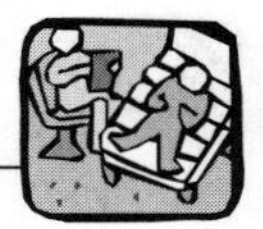

OSCE 30

Instructions for candidate

Assess this tearful woman who gave birth a few weeks ago. Explain the diagnosis and the treatment to this patient.

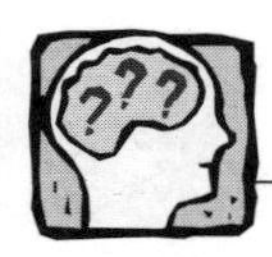

Instructions for actor

You are a 27-year-old woman who has just given birth to her first baby. It was a planned pregnancy, and there were no problems during either the pregnancy or labour. However, for the past couple of weeks since the birth of your daughter you have been feeling very tearful and low in mood. You have been finding it difficult to look after the baby, and you feel that you are a bad mother. Increasingly you find yourself to be very irritable, tired and crying all the time. Before the delivery you were very enthusiastic about the pregnancy, but at present you are not sure how you feel towards your daughter, and this has made you feel guilty. Your husband works shifts and has been away quite often recently.

You have been depressed once in the past. On that occasion you took an antidepressant for about six months.

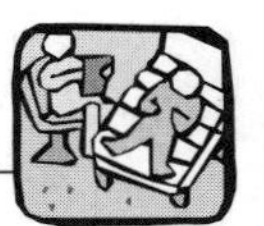

Construct

The candidate should be able to demonstrate a good understanding of puerperal disorders, and to assess the risk to the mother and the baby. They also need to explain the diagnosis and management plan to the patient.

Examiner's marking sheet

	Excellent	Good	Satisfactory	Fail	Poor
Communication skills					
Establishing a diagnosis of postnatal depression					
Assessment of risk to the patient and/or the baby					
Ability to answer the patient's questions					
Overall mark					

Communication skills

You need to establish a good rapport with this woman and be tactful when asking questions. This is quite a sensitive issue for the mother, as she is feeling very vulnerable and is unsure of her feelings towards her baby. It is important to be considerate at all times, and to be very empathetic in your questioning style.

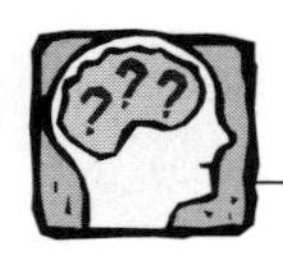

You should be able to answer the questions that the mother is likely to ask and quell any anxieties that she might have about her condition. To score high marks it is essential to avoid the use of jargon and technical terms.

You should introduce yourself and explain the purpose of the interview so as to put the patient at ease and develop a good rapport.

Establishing a diagnosis of post-natal depression

It is essential to establish a diagnosis of depression in this scenario. It is also crucial to demonstrate to the examiner, by your questioning, the difference between postnatal depression and post-partum blues. Next you should rule out the presence of any psychotic symptoms, which if present would be likely to increase the risk both to your patient and to the baby.

Assessment of risk to the patient and/or the baby

This part of the OSCE will be weighted heavily and the examiner will be looking out for your competence in risk assessment, which needs to be undertaken in a proficient and empathetic manner.

Always remember when assessing risk to consider the two domains of **risk to self** and **risk to others**.

Risk to self

This can be due to self-harm behaviour or harm due to self-neglect. You could ask the following:

> 'When people are stressed or feeling low they often get thoughts of wanting to harm themselves. Have you ever had such thoughts?'

Risk to others

In this case we are mainly concerned about the welfare of the baby. This topic needs to be broached gently with the patient, as it is often a source of great anxiety to the mother that she has thoughts that might endanger her baby. Mothers are often relieved when these feelings and emotions are discussed freely with them.

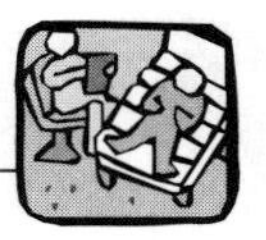

You can gently probe the possibility of risk to the baby by asking a very general question. For example:

> 'How are things with your baby? Have you been coping?'

or

> 'It must be hard with a new baby?'

The use of such normalising questions will put the patient at ease and you will be more likely to elicit a good history. Usually this general approach should be followed by more direct questioning to ascertain the thoughts of the patient. For example:

> 'Have there been times when you wished that your baby wasn't there, or when you have been having a bad day, have you had thoughts of wanting to do anything to your baby?'

It is important to reassure the patient and encourage her to talk freely at every stage of the interview. For example:

> 'I know it is probably quite difficult for you to talk.'

In this scenario the actor will have been instructed to ask you some questions about the doubts she may have concerning the diagnosis or certain aspects of her treatment.

The actress has been primed to ask a number of questions

What is wrong with me? Why am I feeling like this?

The patient needs reassurance that she is suffering from a condition known as postnatal depression. You should emphasise that it is quite common after childbirth, and affects one in ten women.

Why does it happen? Am I going mad?

You should reassure the patient that this is a very treatable condition and that there are several factors which might play a role in contributing to the condition, rather than there being a single cause.

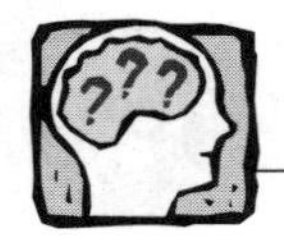

Some of the risk factors include the following:

- previous history of depression
- lack of support
- other financial and social causes of stress.

What about treatment? What do I need?

You should explain to the patient that there is a wide variety of sources of support and treatment available to her. Explain to her that she will receive help in the form of medication (antidepressants), supportive counselling and regular follow-up and support in the community. You should also give her information about voluntary organisations that can provide her with support and useful information about her condition.

Further reading

Royal College of Psychiatrists. *Postnatal depression – help is at hand*; www.rcpsych.ac.uk/info/help/pndep/index_printable.htm

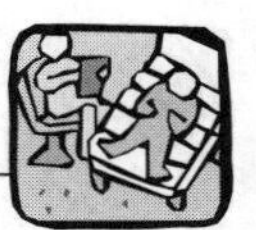

OSCE 31

Instructions for candidate

Give a brief explanation of psychodynamic psychotherapy to this patient who has been suffering from recurrent depressive disorder.

Instructions for actor

You are a 38-year-old woman who has a long history of recurrent depressive disorder. Over the past ten years or so you have been on several antidepressants. For the past year your current treatment plan has not seemed to be relieving your symptoms. There are still days when you are tearful and low in mood, and for the last two months things have been getting worse. Your consultant has just offered to refer you to a psychotherapist for psychodynamic psychotherapy. You are not sure whether this treatment is for you.

You should ask the following questions:

1 How does the treatment work?

2 Does it have any side-effects?

3 Will I need to take my tablets as well?

4 For how long will I need to have therapy?

5 What if the treatment makes me worse or there is an emergency?

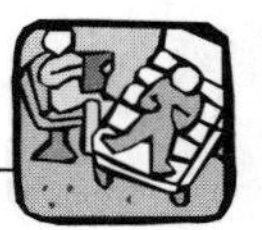

Construct

The candidate should be able to demonstrate a good understanding of the principles of psychodynamic psychotherapy and to explain how it would help the patient. At the same time they should be reassuring and empathise with the patient.

Examiner's marking sheet

	Excellent	Good	Satisfactory	Fail	Poor
Communication skills					
Explanation of the basic principles of and indications for psychodynamic psychotherapy					
Explanation of the nature and process of therapy					
Explanation of the benefits and side-effects of treatment					
Overall mark					

Communication skills

In this OSCE your communication skills are being tested above all else. Your role is not only to explain the process of psychotherapy to the patient, but also to be reassuring and understanding. The actor may have been instructed to be very sceptical and negative about the treatment that has been offered to her, so it is important to be able to demonstrate confidently your knowledge of the subject. If

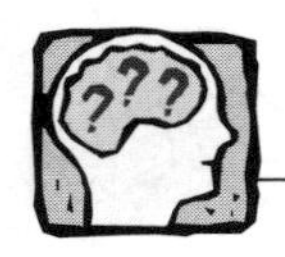

she challenges your views, you should note and acknowledge this, but you should not be tempted to become confrontational.

After you have introduced yourself and explained your role to the patient, you should describe to her the purpose of the interview. If at any stage in the exam you feel that you are running out of time, reassure the patient that you will discuss her queries in more detail later on.

To pass this OSCE you will need to explain the basis principles of and indications for psychodynamic psychotherapy to the patient. Also describe the nature and process of therapy along with the benefits and side-effects of treatment.

Explanation of the basic principles of and indications for psychodynamic psychotherapy

You should explain to the patient that psychodynamic psychotherapy is a form of 'talking treatment'. It is usually indicated in conditions such as depression, and it should help to improve her symptoms.

One of the basic principles of psychodynamic psychotherapy is the exploration of past conflicts and relationships. The relationship between the therapist and the client is paramount with regard to understanding some of the conflicts that the patient may be experiencing, or that they have experienced in the past.

Explanation of the nature and process of therapy

The patient will be very eager to know how the therapy is delivered and over what time-frame. You should explain that the number of sessions will be decided after an initial assessment by the therapist to determine whether this form of therapy would be suitable for the patient. The duration of treatment can vary from just a few months to years, depending on whether it is brief or long-term psychodynamic psychotherapy. You should explain that the sessions are for fixed times and that it is important not to miss any sessions without giving prior notice.

It is important to assure the patient that all other treatment and support will continue unchanged during the period of therapy.

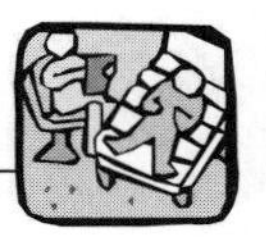

Explanation of the benefits and side-effects of treatment

You should reassure the patient that psychotherapy does not have 'side-effects' in the sense that medication does. However, it does not help everyone and in some cases, especially during the early stages of treatment, it may make the patient feel worse as it involves looking at some of the past relationships and trauma that she might have experienced. You should also explain that one of the benefits of psychotherapy is that it is long-lasting and will be effective in improving both her symptoms and how she interacts with other people.

Further reading

Wright, P., Stern, J. and Phelan, M. 2000. *Core psychiatry*. W.B. Saunders.

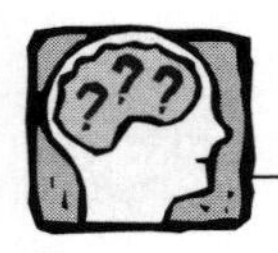

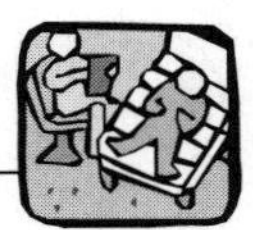

OSCE 32

Instructions for candidate

Perform a neurological examination of the lower limbs of this patient, giving a running commentary as you do so.

Construct

The candidate should be able to demonstrate a good understanding of how to conduct a neurological examination. Their approach should be systematic, showing consideration to the patient at all times. Clear instructions should be given to the patient.

Examiner's marking sheet

	Excellent	Good	Satisfactory	Fail	Poor
Communication skills					
General examination and inspection					
Examination of the tone and power of muscle groups					
Examination of reflexes					
Examination of co-ordination					
Overall mark					

Communication skills

When you have introduced yourself to the patient, it is important to explain to them what you are about to do, and in particular to obtain their permission before you start. Always be courteous and avoid causing any discomfort to the patient. If you think that any procedure may cause some degree of discomfort, forewarn them about it.

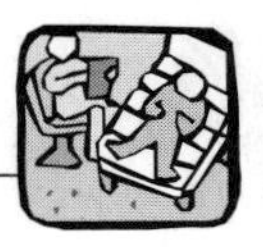

Examine the patient systematically, giving a clear commentary to the examiner about what you are doing (a similar approach should be used if examination of the upper limb is required). The examination should be performed under the following headings.

Important tip: Make use of all the equipment provided at this OSCE station for your examination.

General examination and inspection

Neurological examination of the lower limbs

Before you start, ask the patient whether they have any pain or discomfort in the lower limbs.

Inspection

Look for any asymmetry of the limbs. Is there any evidence of muscle wasting either proximally or distally? Look for any fasciculations and deformity in the legs and feet.

Clonus needs to be tested.

Gait

Your examination will not be complete unless you comment on the gait of the patient. Be alert for an unsteady gait, a limp, foot-drop or arm-swing.

Sensory system

The main sensory modalities that should be tested are as follows:

- pinprick – this tests superficial pain
- vibration sense (across the ankle, knee and pelvis)
- joint position – this tests proprioception (big toe and ankle)
- light touch – this should be tested last.

Examination of the tone and power of muscle groups

Tone

This can be tested by either rolling the leg on the bed or by flexing and extending the knee.

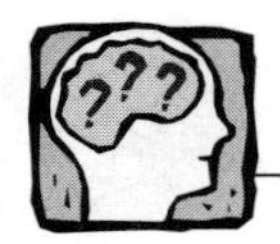

Power

The power of the various muscle groups must be tested across all major joints. The power needs to be rated using the MRC power scale as follows:

0 = no movement
1 = just a flicker of muscle movement
2 = movement with gravity eliminated
3 = movement against gravity but not against resistance
4 = movement against resistance, but not normal power
5 = normal power.

You will need to know the myotomes across these joints when you are testing the power of the groups of muscles.

Hip adduction L_1-L_3
Hip abduction L_3
Hip flexion L_3, L_4
Hip extension L_4, L_5

Knee flexion L_4, L_5
Knee extension L_3, L_4
Dorsiflexion of foot L_5
Plantar flexion of foot S_1

Examination of reflexes

The reflexes that are normally tested are the knee jerk (L_3, L_4), ankle reflex (L_5, S_1) and plantar response.

Knee jerk

To demonstrate this, lift the patient's knees to 20 degrees of flexion by supporting them with your arm. Then tap the patellar tendon and watch for the quadriceps muscle contracting with the knee extending.

Ankle jerk

To demonstrate this, have the hip and knee slightly flexed with one hand grasping the forefoot. Then allow the hammer to strike the Achilles tendon and watch for plantar flexion and calf muscle contraction.

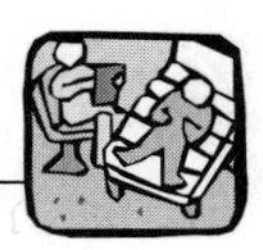

Plantar response

Explain to the patient that you have to scrape the bottom of their foot with the sharp end of the tendon hammer. Scrape with the sharp end from the outside of the foot, starting from the heel and working upwards and then across the forefoot.

Note: The normal response is for the big toe and the other toes to show plantar flexion (ie downward motion).

Examination of co-ordination

Co-ordination should be tested last, as it requires an intact motor and sensory system. In the lower limb the following can be used to check co-ordination:

- heel-shin test
- walking in a straight line
- Romberg's test – ask the patient to stand with their feet together and their eyes closed. If the patient sways to one side, this indicates posterior column degeneration.

Further reading

Macleod, J., Munro, J.F. and Campbell, I. 2000. *Macleod's clinical examination*. Churchill Livingstone.

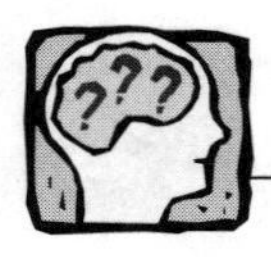

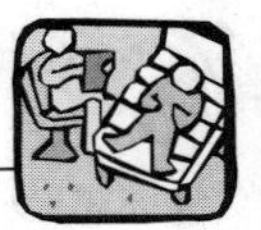

OSCE 33

Instructions for candidate

Elicit a history of psychosis from this 30-year-old man who has been brought to the Accident and Emergency department by his partner. The partner reports that the patient has been behaving abnormally for the past two weeks and during that time has become more paranoid and hostile.

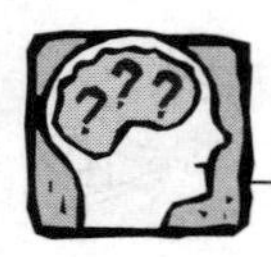

Instructions for actor

You are a 30-year-old man who has been brought to the Accident and Emergency department by your partner. You have been smoking cannabis excessively for the past two weeks. During that time you have been feeling very paranoid, and you believe that there is a conspiracy against you. You feel that because of your special ability to read the minds of other people you are wanted by the Government. For the past couple of days you have been staying in your flat and not going out. You have not had any other abnormal experiences. You are generally healthy and have never had any psychiatric or medical problems.

At present you are smoking cannabis every day, as this helps to relax you, especially since you lost your job as a salesman last week.

You are generally irritable during the interview and do not disclose any information unless specifically asked to do so by the candidate.

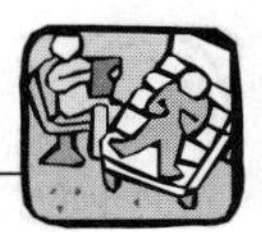

Construct

This OSCE assesses the candidate's ability to take a relevant history and perform a mental state examination with a view to demonstrating abnormal perceptions and thoughts. The candidate should be able to demonstrate the obvious psychopathology and at the same time rule out any other significant abnormalities. They should also show that they are able both to control the interview and to gain the confidence and trust of the patient.

Examiner's marking sheet

	Excellent	Good	Satisfactory	Fail	Poor
Communication skills					
Obtaining a brief relevant history					
Establishing the relevant psychopathology					
Assessment of risk					
Overall mark					

Communication skills

One of the main aspects that is being assessed in this OSCE is ability to control the interview and take a relevant history from an agitated patient. One of the most important things to remember when you are faced with a difficult patient is the need to establish and then build rapport with them. Therefore you must avoid moving straight into direct questioning of the patient's condition, and instead start with some open and general questioning.

Set the scene by introducing yourself and explaining your role and the purpose of your interview.

Obtaining a brief relevant history

As stated above, one of the key tasks in this scenario is to establish good rapport and demonstrate ability to control the interview. Next it is vital for you to take a basic background history that covers past psychiatric history, family history and, most importantly, drug and alcohol history. Details are not essential, but this brief history will provide you with clues to the underlying diagnosis.

Establishing the relevant psychopathology

The next step is to perform a thorough mental state examination. Remember that at this stage you have not made a diagnosis, so it is important to rule out all of the possibilities and to screen for all likely conditions, including affective disorders.

Establishing the presence of delusions

The mental state examination should be carried out under all of the usual headings, but here we shall focus on how you can elicit psychotic symptoms. It is quite easy to miss a history of psychosis, especially if the patient is speaking coherently and has a good grasp of reality. Therefore it is helpful to start with some general screening questions for psychotic symptoms. For example:

> 'Have you had any strange or odd experiences lately that you can't explain?'

> 'Do you ever hear or see things that other people can't hear or see?'

Although this is a more direct line of questioning, it is easier for the patient to understand and preferable to asking, for example, 'Do you hear voices?' – to which the patient might answer 'yes', thinking that you are asking about his hearing.

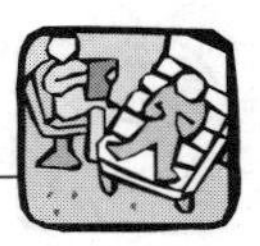

Once you have established that the patient has some psychotic features, it is important to confirm the nature of the symptoms.

Persecutory delusions
You could enquire about these by asking the following questions:

'Have you had trouble getting along with people?'

'Has anyone been trying to harm you in any way?'

The patient may have isolated beliefs of persecution, or these beliefs may be very systematised and involve all facets of their life.

Grandiose delusions
Here the patient believes that they have special powers. You can elicit these delusions by asking the following questions:

'Do you feel special in any way?'

'Do you think that you have special powers, talents or abilities?'

'Do you feel that you are going to achieve great things?'

Religious delusions
It is important to obtain background information about the patient's belief system. You could begin by asking the following questions:

'Are you a religious person?'

'Have you had any religious experiences recently?'

Remember that the interpretation of a person's beliefs depends upon their cultural and religious background.

Delusions or ideas of reference
Here the patient believes that events around them have special personal significance and are referring to them. You can elicit a delusion of reference by asking the following questions:

'Do you ever get the feeling when you walk into a room that people were talking about you or laughing at you?'

'Have you seen things in the newspaper or on television that seem to talk about you or contain a special message for you?'

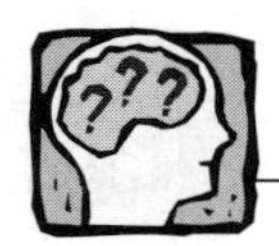

Somatic delusions

Here the patient believes that their body is diseased, abnormal or changed. The following are good screening questions for eliciting somatic delusions:

> 'Is there anything wrong with the way your body is working?'
>
> 'Have you noticed any change in your appearance?'

Next it is vital to rule out the presence of any first-rank symptoms of schizophrenia (for guidance on the type of questions to ask, see OSCE 26).

Establishing the presence of abnormal perceptions

You need to elicit first-rank auditory hallucinations (for details of how to do this, see OSCE 26) and also to rule out the presence of other types of abnormal perceptions, such as somatic or tactile, olfactory and visual hallucinations.

Somatic or tactile hallucinations

These involve abnormal bodily experiences. You can begin by questioning the patient as follows:

> 'Have you had any strange feelings in your body?'

If they give a positive response, ask them to elaborate.

Olfactory hallucinations

These are often confused with abnormal smells. Question the patient as follows:

> 'Have you experienced any odd or unusual smells or tastes recently that others did not notice?'

Visual hallucinations

The patient may describe seeing shapes or people that are not actually present. In an acute state he or she may even be responding to them. You can elicit visual hallucinations by observing the patient and questioning them as follows:

> 'Have you seen things that other people cannot see?'

Follow this up by asking: 'What did you see?'

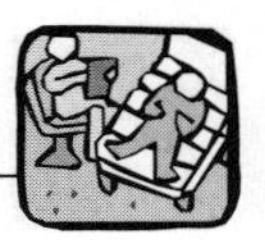

Assessment of risk

After screening for psychosis and asking the relevant questions, do not forget to screen for differential diagnoses or affective disorders. It is important that you then highlight to the examiner the importance of gauging what this patient's current risk is both to himself and to others.

Remember that this OSCE scenario is a time-consuming one. It is therefore essential to be methodical when assessing such a patient, so that you do not overlook the essentials.

Further reading

Andreasen, N.C. and Black, D.W. 2001. *Introductory textbook of psychiatry*, third edn. American Psychiatric Publishing Inc., pp59-67.

Carlat, J.D. 1999. *The psychiatric interview*. Lippincott Williams & Wilkins, pp183-200.

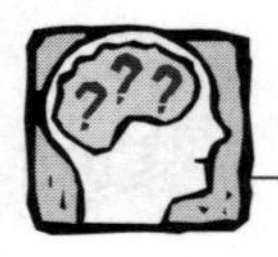

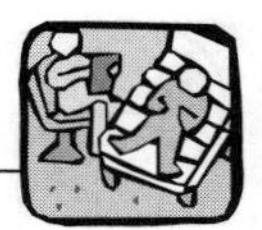

OSCE 34

Instructions for candidate

Discuss the initiation of lithium therapy with this 30-year-old woman. Address the patient's concerns, beliefs and expectations with regard to the treatment.

Instructions for actor

You are a 30-year-old woman who has been diagnosed with bipolar affective disorder. The consultant has suggested that you should start lithium therapy. You are quite anxious about the treatment, and have asked to see the senior house officer to discuss some of your concerns.

You ask the following questions:

1. For how long will I need treatment?
2. Is the treatment associated with any side-effects?
3. I have heard that I need blood tests. Why do I need these tests?
4. I am thinking of having a baby soon. Will there be any problems with that?

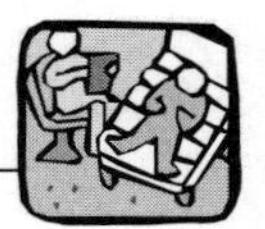

Construct

This OSCE assesses the candidate's ability to communicate their knowledge of lithium therapy to the patient in simple language, with empathy and understanding of the patient's needs.

Examiner's marking sheet

	Excellent	Good	Satisfactory	Fail	Poor
Communication skills					
Explanation of the indications for lithium					
Explanation of the side-effects of lithium					
Explanation of the need for blood tests					
Ability to answer the patient's questions					
Overall mark					

Communication skills

You are very likely to encounter this OSCE, and you need to be well versed in all of the indications for and side-effects of lithium. Importantly, if the patient is a young woman, you must be prepared to advise her on pregnancy and breastfeeding. A key component of this station is communication, and you will score high marks if you can explain lithium treatment and its side-effects in simple, jargon-free language.

Start by introducing yourself and explaining your role and the purpose of the interview. After obtaining brief background information about the patient, you should cover each of the following areas.

Explanation of the indications for lithium

First you need to clarify with the patient what she knows about the treatment. Explain to her that lithium is a naturally occurring substance and that it is widely used for the treatment of bipolar disorders. You should emphasise that it is a very effective form of treatment for her condition.

Explanation of the side-effects of lithium

The side-effects should be described in a simple and succinct manner. You should explain that the patient can expect to experience side-effects within the first week of treatment, but that they do improve over time.

It is important to list some of the common side-effects of lithium, which include the following:

- feeling thirsty
- passing more urine
- fine tremor in the hands
- weight gain
- occasionally, blurring of vision.

You need to make it clear to the patient that if she experiences any of the following toxic symptoms she must get in touch with her doctor:

- vomiting or severe diarrhoea
- staggering or unstable gait
- slurred speech.

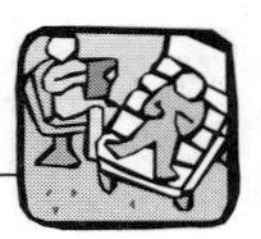

Explanation of the need for blood tests

Blood tests are crucial to the safe prescribing of lithium. You must explain to the patient that initially she will need blood tests every few weeks, until her lithium levels are adequate. You should emphasise that she will need the tests for as long as she is on lithium, but that the frequency of the tests will decrease. In addition, she will require regular monitoring of her thyroid and renal function.

The actress has been primed to ask a number of questions

Explanation of treatment in relation to pregnancy and breastfeeding

This is an important area and the patient will be quite anxious to have her questions answered, to put her mind at ease. You must explain to her that if she does become pregnant, it is usually better to stop the lithium. However, this needs to be done after consultation with her psychiatrist, who will consider putting her on alternative medication. With regard to breastfeeding you must make it absolutely clear that the patient cannot breastfeed while she is on lithium, as the drug passes into the breast milk.

Discussion of additional support available to patient

Reassure the patient that she is not alone in her battle against her illness. She can receive plenty of support and help not only from her GP, psychiatrist and community psychiatric nurse, but also from voluntary organisations such as the Manic Depression Fellowship (www.mdf.org.uk). You could tell her that you will collect more information and pass it on to her.

Note: It is perfectly acceptable for you to say in the exam that you will arrange another appointment to see the patient again if she has any other queries about her treatment. This is a good conclusion that you can use for most OSCE stations.

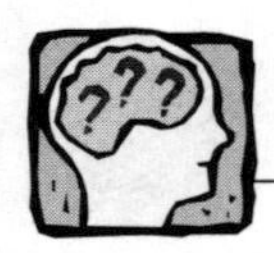

Further reading

Royal College of Psychiatrists. *Manic-depressive illness*, patient fact sheet; www.rcpsych.ac.uk/info/help/manicdep/index.htm

Taylor, D., Paton, C. and Kerwin, R. 2003. *Prescribing guidelines*, 7th edn. Martin Dunitz, pp93–96.

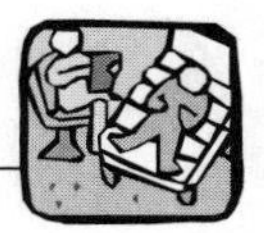

OSCE 35

Instructions for candidate

Take a history from this patient with somatisation disorder or unexplained medical symptoms.

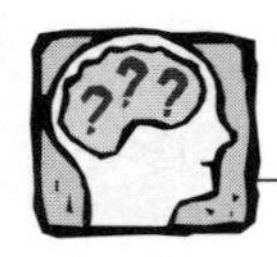

Instructions for actor

You are a 25-year-old housewife who has been referred to the psychiatrist by the consultant physician. For the last two years you have been experiencing weakness and malaise. You have also been experiencing burning pain in your eyes, and muscular aches in your back, neck, and upper and lower limbs. For the past six to eight months you have also been experiencing severe nausea and vomiting. You have been to see a gastroenterologist about these symptoms, but several investigations revealed nothing conclusive.

Prior to this you were in hospital, when you were investigated for repeated blackouts and dizzy spells. More recently you have been having heavy periods and bloating of your lower abdomen. You have been seeing a gynaecologist about these symptoms.

In the past you have had several investigations for your thyroid, and you have experienced recurrent abdominal pain. You have also had some surgery, which included an appendicectomy.

You are not sure why you are in a psychiatric outpatient clinic, and you think that someone has made an error in referring you here.

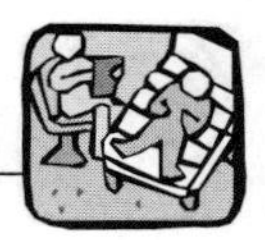

Construct

This OSCE assesses the candidate's ability to reassure and empathise with the patient, who has little psychological understanding of her condition. Also being tested is the candidate's ability to take a relevant history to allow them to make a diagnosis. The candidate should demonstrate that they can gain the confidence of an angry patient.

Examiner's marking sheet

	Excellent	Good	Satisfactory	Fail	Poor
Communication skills					
Obtaining a history relevant to making a diagnosis					
Ruling out other possible psychiatric conditions					
Brief assessment of risk					
Overall mark					

Note: Somatisation has been used as a descriptive term for patients who have a tendency to manifest psychological and interpersonal distress in the form of somatic distress and medically unexplained symptoms for which they seek medical help.

Communication skills

Communication is a key element in this scenario. You need to gain the confidence of your patient so that she is able to narrate a good

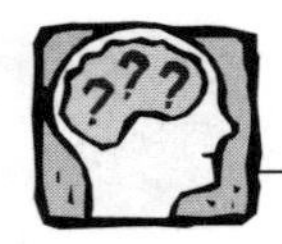

history. Introduce yourself and then explain your role and the reasons for the interview.

You need to explain to the patient that your role as a psychiatrist is to find out whether there are other reasons or explanations for her symptoms. You need to reassure her that there may be other alternative approaches to help her with some of the problems she has been facing. Many patients who are seeing a psychiatrist for the first time fear that they will be labelled as a 'nutter'. You need to encourage the patient to speak to you and reassure her that this will not be the case.

Once you have established a rapport with the patient, you need to obtain a history relevant to making a diagnosis, rule out other possible psychiatric conditions, and make a brief risk assessment.

Obtaining a history relevant to making a diagnosis

To make a diagnosis of somatisation disorder you will have to demonstrate the following in this patient:

- a history of many physical complaints, beginning before the age of 30 years, that have occurred over a period of several years
- impairment of social, occupational or other important areas of functioning.

To make a diagnosis you should also elicit from the patient a history of the following:

- pain at four different sites
- at least two gastrointestinal symptoms (eg nausea, vomiting, bloating)
- at least one sexual or reproductive symptom (eg irregular menses, erectile or ejaculatory problems)
- one pseudoneurological symptom (eg paralysis, problems with balance, swallowing difficulties)

You should also establish that even after appropriate investigations have been performed the above symptoms cannot be accounted for by a known general medical condition. It is equally important to establish that if a general medical condition has been diagnosed, the symptoms and disabilities are out of proportion to the underlying pathology.

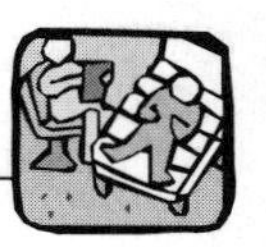

Finally, you should ascertain whether these symptoms are being produced or feigned intentionally (as in a factitious disorder). The above guidance is based on DSM-IV criteria for diagnosing somatisation disorder. Whether you use ICD-10 or DSM-IV criteria for making a diagnosis, make sure that you are methodical and cover all areas.

Ruling out other possible psychiatric conditions

This is a key part of your history taking. You need to ensure that the patient is not suffering from an underlying depression or any other serious mental illness. You will therefore have to screen for depression and psychosis with the relevant questions. A common association is with substance misuse and dependence, so it is equally important to screen for drugs and alcohol in your history taking.

Brief assessment of risk

You must ensure that there are no underlying risk factors, such as risk of deliberate self-harm or suicide.

A good general way to conclude this station is to offer to see the patient again, when you will discuss with her in more detail some of the issues that you have covered today.

Further reading

Andreasen, N.C. and Black, D.W. 2001. *Introductory textbook of psychiatry*, 3rd edn. American Psychiatric Publishing Inc., pp363–370.

Wise, G.M. and Rundell, J.R. 2002. *Textbook of consultation liaison psychiatry*, 2nd edn. American Psychiatric Publishing, pp361–367.

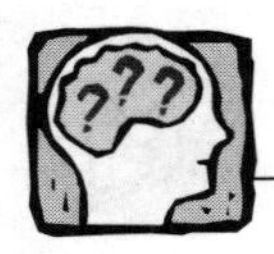

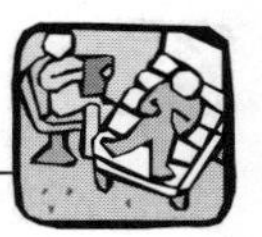

OSCE 36

Instructions for candidate

Explain to this patient, who has been diagnosed with schizophrenia and has recently been started on antipsychotic treatment, why he cannot drive.

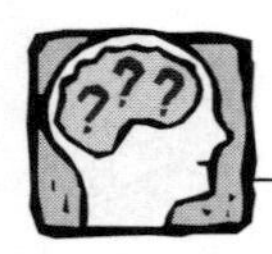

Instructions for actor

You are a 28-year-old man who has recently been diagnosed with schizophrenia, and you have been started on treatment with olanzapine, an antipsychotic. You have been doing well for the past four months since you have been discharged from hospital.

At present you are living with your parents and you have been depending on them to drive you everywhere. However, you are planning to move out as you have recently found a job. You have come for an outpatient follow-up appointment and are keen to start driving again as soon as possible.

You ask the following questions:

1. Is it possible for me to start driving?
2. What do I have to do next before I can start driving?
3. Will my insurance be affected?

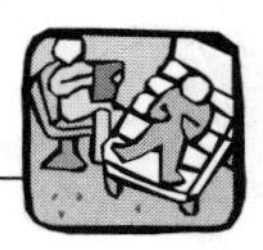

Construct

This OSCE assesses the candidate's communication skills and their ability to demonstrate a good understanding of the regulations concerning driving after a psychotic illness. They should empathise with the patient's needs and concerns.

Examiner's marking sheet

	Excellent	Good	Satisfactory	Fail	Poor
Communication skills					
Examination of reflexes					
Examination of co-ordination					
Discussion of the issues relating to driving					
Overall mark					

Communication skills

The patient is obviously quite concerned about his driving and the implications of his ability to drive. You must be patient and empathise with these concerns. Be reassuring and polite, as the patient is likely to become frustrated when he realises that he will have to wait until he hears the decision of the DVLA concerning his driving.

Introduce yourself and explain your role and the purpose of the interview. Early on you should clarify what the patient's expectations are, so that you can deal with them as you go along.

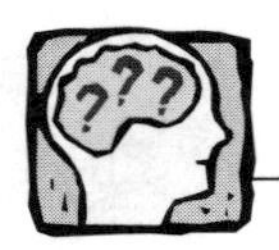

After covering the patient's background briefly you need to focus on the main task, which is to address the issues of driving and antipsychotic medication. You also need to examine the patient's reflexes and co-ordination.

Discussion of the issues relating to driving

Explanation of the relationship between driving and antipsychotic medication

You need to explain to the patient that his driving would be impaired as a result of his psychotropic medication. Mention that the medication may impair his co-ordination and response time, and that this could have an impact on his driving ability. Before he can start driving again he needs to inform the DVLA, who will then request a medical assessment.

In the case of patients with an acute psychotic condition the licence is usually revoked for at least 12 months. With regard to chronic schizophrenia, driving is usually permitted in the case of patients who have been stable and had no relapses in the past 12 months.

Explanation of the duty of the patient

You need to explain clearly that it is the patient's responsibility to inform the Drivers Medical Unit at the DVLA if they develop a new medical condition, or if a current medical condition has worsened since their driving licence was issued.

Explanation to the patient of the duty of the prescriber

You must maintain the patient's right to confidentiality at all times. However, if you feel that the patient does not have capacity or is not heeding your advice on driving, you have a duty to inform the DVLA about this breach by your patient. There is no discretion on this subject, and the situation must be made clear to the patient.

Further reading

DVLA. *Psychiatric conditions and driving at a glance*; www.dvla.gov.uk/at_a_glance/ch4_psychiatric.htm

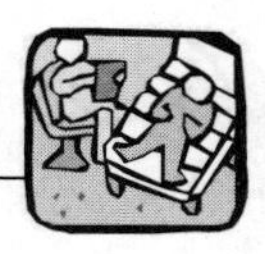

Metzner, J.L., Dentino, A.N. and Goddard, S.L. 1993. Impairment in driving and psychiatric illness. *Journal of Neuropsychiatry*, 5, 211–220.

Taylor, D., Paton, C. and Kerwin, R. 2003. *Prescribing guidelines*, 7th edn. Martin Dunitz, pp255–259.

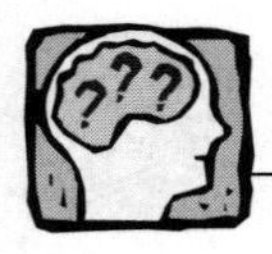

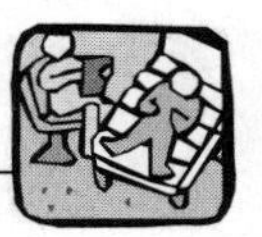

OSCE 37

Instructions for candidate

You have been asked to see a 28-year-old man with a diagnosis of schizophrenia who has been treated with olanzapine 15 mg for the past two years. He has been doing well and is living independently.

You are seeing him in the clinic because of the problems he has been having with weight gain since starting the medication. Assess the patient and give him some practical advice about this problem.

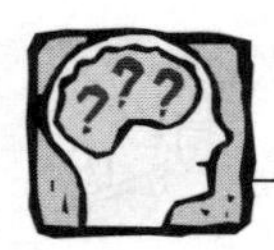

Instructions for actor

You are 28-year-old man with a history of schizophrenia. You are currently taking olanzapine. You have been doing well except for the fact that for the past year or so you have put on more than two stones in weight. You are very concerned about this. With regard to your mental state this is the best you have ever been.

Ask the following questions:

1. What is causing the weight gain?
2. What can I do to help myself?
3. Would an alternative medication be of any help?

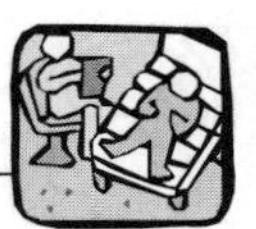

Construct

In this OSCE the candidate has to demonstrate that they have good communication skills – that is, they are able to develop a good rapport with the patient and put him at ease so that he is able to discuss his problem freely. It is equally important that the candidate is able to explain to the patient the reasons for his problem in plain and simple language.

Examiner's marking sheet

	Excellent	Good	Satisfactory	Fail	Poor
Communication skills					
Thorough relevant background history					
Ability to give helpful practical advice on medication and lifestyle					
Overall mark					

Communication skills

High marks in this station are dependent on your communication style. The subject matter is simple, but you need to be able to clarify the patient's concerns and also give him some practical advice.

Set the scene in the usual manner by introducing yourself and explaining the purpose of the interview. Establish at the outset what the patient's concerns are and how you may be able to help him.

Thorough relevant background history

It is important to spend a few minutes gathering some background information about factors that might be contributing to the patient's presentation, so that you can give sound and relevant advice. You need to obtain a brief medical history to establish whether the patient has any other risk factors, including a list of current medication. You also need to have some idea of the patient's lifestyle and level of activity.

Ability to give helpful practical advice on medication and lifestyle

It is important to explain to the patient that one of the common problems with all antipsychotic drugs is that they can cause weight gain. The weight gain does vary from one person to another and also from one drug to another. However, what has to be emphasised is that we need to balance the pros and the cons of taking the medication, and that there are more benefits from taking the medication than there are drawbacks. Furthermore, at present there is little evidence to support the view that switching antipsychotics will necessarily cause a weight reduction.

You need to empathise with the patient and acknowledge that weight gain is socially disabling as well as being an important risk factor for various medical conditions, including heart disease.

You should explain to the patient that there are plenty of ways to help him to lose weight. Advise him on his dietary intake and encourage him to gradually increase his level of physical activity. Explain to him that he needs to have a well-balanced diet that includes plenty of fruit and vegetables. You could also tell him that you will refer him to a nutritionist who can give him more specific advice on calories and look at specific aspects of his dietary intake.

The message that needs to be reinforced is 'Eat a little less and exercise a little more'.

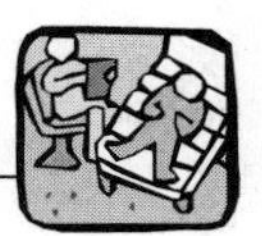

Further reading

Pendelbury, J. and Ost, D. 2002. *Cromwell House weight management programme for patients with severe enduring mental illness: preliminary results.* Poster presented at ECNP (European College of Neuropsychopharmacology) Annual Congress, Barcelona, Spain, 5–9 October 2002.

Taylor, D., Paton, C. and Kerwin, R. 2003. *Prescribing guidelines*, 7th edn. Martin Dunitz, pp72–73.

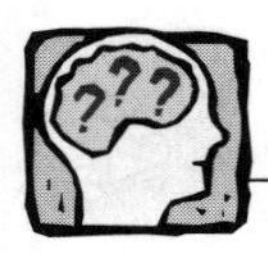

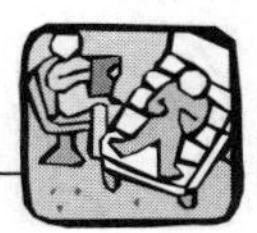

OSCE 38

Instructions for candidate

A patient has attended the clinic for his regular depot medication. His usual community psychiatric nurse is unavailable, and you have been asked to cover. Using the equipment provided, with the cushion provided as a model for the patient's buttock, demonstrate how you would inject the depot. Provide the examiners with an explanation for your method as you proceed.

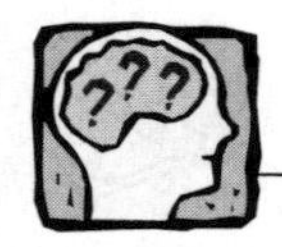

Equipment provided

- Cushion – labelled with the name of the 'patient'
- Syringes and needles in a range of sizes
- 1 mL ampoule labelled 'zuclopenthixol decanoate 200 mg/mL'
- 1 mL ampoule labelled 'zuclopenthixol acetate 50 mg/mL'
- Paper towel
- Drug chart written up for '150 mg Clopixol im depot' due today
- Steri-wipe
- Piece of cotton wool
- Plaster
- Sharps bin
- Bucket/sink.

Construct

This OSCE assesses the candidate's practical skills and knowledge with regard to the safe administration of medicines in general, and the deep intramuscular injection of depot neuroleptic in particular.

Examiner's marking sheet

	Excellent	Good	Satisfactory	Fail	Poor
Administration of medicines					
Injection technique					
Explanation					
Overall mark					

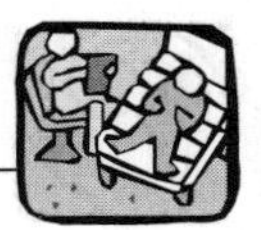

Commentary

You should first inspect the drug chart, checking the patient ID, the drug and the date. Then select the correct ampoule (labelled zuclopenthixol decanoate 200 mg/mL), an appropriate size of syringe (2.5 mL) to achieve an accurate measurement, and an appropriate gauge of needle (at least green) to effectively draw up the oily depot.

You should break the ampoule, preferably using the paper towel to avoid injury, discard the top of the ampoule in the sharps bin, draw up the contents into the syringe, and discard the remainder of the ampoule safely. The excess drug should be expelled into the sink while you hold the syringe at eye level to ensure precision. The volume remaining in the syringe should be 0.75 mL.

The first needle should then be discarded as a sharp (since it has now been blunted) and replaced with a second needle (which should be green) that is small enough to minimise pain on injection but not so small that you run the risk of poor penetration and/or breakage.

Before injection, the intended site should be swabbed and tensed – to enable so-called 'Z'-tracking between the different skin layers, thereby promoting haemostasis.

Note: In the case of a real patient or actor the site should be selected only after you have reviewed the notes, consulted the patient and inspected the site, to ensure rotation of the site and so avoid trauma. You will gain marks for mentioning this.

Entry of the needle should be swift but controlled to minimise discomfort. Draw back to avoid intravenous injection, depress the plunger firmly and steadily, withdraw the needle and syringe and place them in the sharps bin, staunch any blood flow with cotton wool, and apply a plaster.

Tips and pointers

As with any test of skill, there is no substitute for practice. In terms of exam technique it is also worth practising giving an explanation of what you are doing while you are doing it – which is actually more demanding and therefore a greater test of confidence in both knowledge and skill.

Reading list

Patterson, C. Injection technique: Depot drugs *Nursing Times* 1998, 25 Nov, 94 (47).

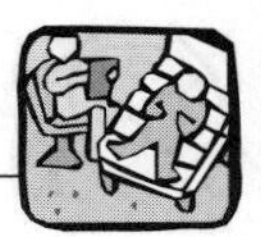

OSCE 39

Instructions for candidate

You are asked to see the mother of a 21-year-old man with a diagnosis of schizophrenia who has recently been readmitted to hospital with a recurrent episode of acute psychosis. She wishes to know what has caused her son's illness. You have the patient's informed consent to share appropriate information with the mother.

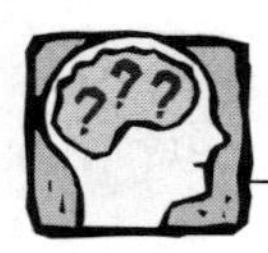

Instructions for actor

This is the second time that your son has been admitted to hospital, and you are becoming increasingly concerned about him and his future. You have recently read in the popular press that cannabis is now considered to be a cause of schizophrenia, which makes you feel very guilty because, as an occasional cannabis smoker yourself, you fear that you may have set a bad example. You have also been told that schizophrenia is due to 'bad blood', which only adds to your anxiety, as you now fear for the health of your other children.

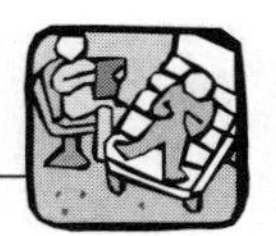

Construct

This OSCE is designed to test a specific area of the candidate's knowledge while at the same time evaluating their general skill in communicating such information to a distressed relative.

Examiner's marking sheet

	Excellent	Good	Satisfactory	Fail	Poor
Communication skills					
Checking boundaries of confidentiality					
Eliciting concerns					
Identifying mother's current level and adequacy of understanding					
Providing appropriate and accurate information communicated in an understandable way					
Instilling reasonable hope and offering further support					
Overall mark					

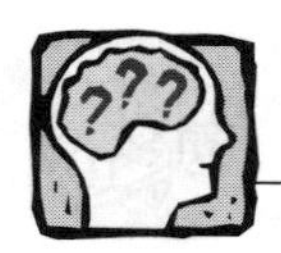

Communication skills and checking boundaries of confidentiality

Once you have established a reasonable rapport, it is important to remember to check the boundaries of confidentiality with any informant. You should explain to the mother:

- that the patient is aware of the meeting and the kind of information that will be passed on, and why
- however, your discussion together is confidential and although it will be noted, its content would not be passed on if sharing that information might be harmful to the patient, the mother or anyone else.

You should check that this is acceptable to the mother before proceeding.

Eliciting concerns and identifying mother's current level of adequacy of understanding

Then, rather than launching into a textbook exposition of the aetiology of schizophrenia, it is important to find out first what concerns the mother has, and more specifically what she already knows and where the gaps or misconceptions are in her knowledge. This will help to match the information you provide to her needs.

Providing appropriate and accurate information communicated in an understandable way

At this stage it is worth pointing out that the precise mechanisms of schizophrenia still remain unclear, and that the diagnosis is used more or less descriptively to define a group of symptoms that include a loss of sense of reality. It is important to add that despite this uncertainty, it is known that effective treatments are available.

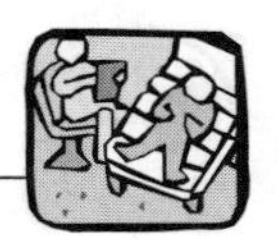

Instilling reasonable hope and offering further support

This will help to instil hope in a relative who may feel overwhelmed by fear. In addressing the mother's specific concerns, you should aim to unburden her of any unnecessary or unhelpful feelings of guilt while at the same time providing accurate information. Exactly how you achieve this will depend to some extent on how the interview proceeds. For example, you could say something similar to the following:

> 'Yes, you are quite right, cannabis is emerging as a potential cause in some cases of schizophrenia' (thereby validating the mother's concern).

You could then add:

> 'However, it is only one cause among many, and it is quite possible that this substance was not a factor in your son's illness. In other words, he may well have developed the illness even if he hadn't used cannabis' (thereby mitigating the mother's guilt).

You could adopt a similar approach to the mother's anxiety about 'bad blood'. Again you should state that the condition has many different causes, including a genetic contribution. However, many cases of schizophrenia do not have a family history, and the risk to family members, and specifically to non-twin siblings, is relatively low (around 10%).

Finally, it is important to offer the mother further opportunities to increase her understanding of her son's condition. These would include a further meeting, written material such as patient information leaflets, referral for a carer's assessment and/or the contact details of local support organisations such as Rethink (www.rethink.org) and MIND (www.mind.org.uk).

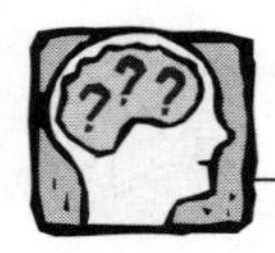

Further reading

National Institute for Clinical Excellence (NICE). 2002. *Treating and managing schizophrenia (core interventions): understanding NICE guidance – information for people with schizophrenia, their advocates and carers, and the public.* London, NICE.

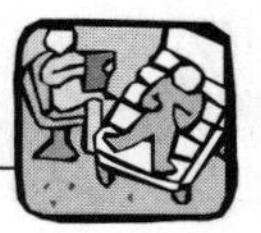

OSCE 40

Instructions for candidate

Please assess this patient for a movement disorder. You are advised to briefly examine the drug chart first. Explain your findings to the patient.

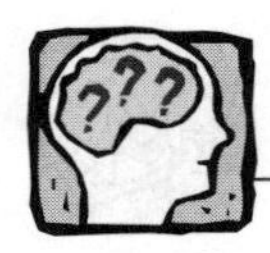

Instructions for actor

You have a feeling of inner restlessness associated with a strong urge to move your legs in an agitated fashion. Consequently, your legs are restless for most of the time. The drug lithium was recently added to your medication regime, but otherwise there have been no changes.

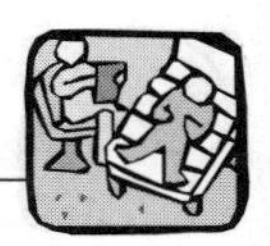

Equipment

- Drug chart written up for Clopixol depot 600 mg weekly and lithium 1 g at night.

Construct

This OSCE is designed to test the candidate's ability to conduct a basic focused neurological examination, and to assess their knowledge of common adverse drug reactions and interactions in psychiatry.

Examiner's marking sheet

	Excellent	Good	Satisfactory	Fail	Poor
Communication skills					
Assessment of movement disorders					
Explanation of movement disorders					
Overall mark					

Communication skills

As instructed, you should consult the drug chart first. The identification of a depot neuroleptic at high dose and in combination with lithium should give you a strong clue – that it is likely you will find evidence of an adverse drug reaction of some kind.

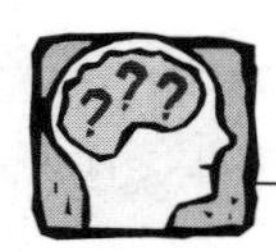

Assessment and knowledge of movement disorders

Note that you are being asked to assess the patient. It is therefore important to be prepared to take a brief history as well as to conduct a focused neurological examination. Ask the patient whether they or anyone else have noticed odd or unusual movements, and ask whether they have any impulse to move in an odd or annoying way. Find out how long the movement has been present, whether it has changed during that time, and what the precipitants (if any) appear to be.

In terms of the examination, you should first inspect the patient at rest. Examine gait, tremor, fine motor co-ordination and tone. If you detect any abnormal movements, ask the patient to attempt to stop these by force of will.

Explanation of movement disorders

Explain to the patient that they have a condition called akathisia or 'restless legs syndrome', which is likely to be due to the medication, namely the injection that they are taking. Tell them that the condition may well have been precipitated by the addition of lithium, a drug which is known to potentiate or enhance the propensity of drugs like Clopixol to cause this kind of side-effect.

For more details on conducting a detailed neurological examination, please see OSCE 32.

Further reading

Pavel Mohr and Jan Volavka, Ladislav Haskovec and Akathisia: 100th anniversary *British Journal of Psychiatry*, December 2002; 181:537

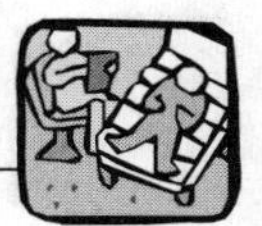

OSCE 41

Instructions for candidate

Examine this patient's mood and then explain your findings to the patient.

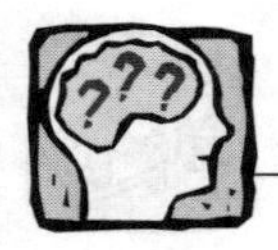

Instructions for actor

You're a 30-year-old woman. You are fed up and angry because you have recently had to work with a new and demanding boss. Meanwhile your partner is complaining that you always come home from work late. Sometimes you lie awake at night for up to an hour worrying about your job, although otherwise your sleep pattern is unchanged.

However, you still enjoy your regular pastimes such as seeing friends and watching your favourite television programmes. Your appetite is good and your weight has remained steady. You feel glad to be alive and think that in general life is good, you have no suicidal ideas, and you continue to enjoy a healthy sexual relationship with your partner.

Someone at work who, like you, is a bit of worrier said that you should try Prozac because it really helped her when she was 'down', so you thought you would check it out.

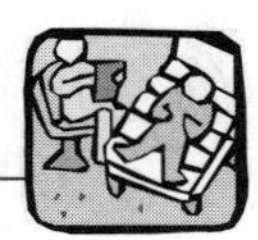

Construct

This OSCE assesses the candidate's ability to discriminate between mental illness and a normal reaction to stress, specifically in relation to depressive-type symptomatology.

Examiner's marking sheet

	Excellent	Good	Satisfactory	Fail	Poor
Communication skills					
Assessment of mood symptoms					
Explanation of findings					
Overall mark					

Communication skills and examination

Once you have established rapport with the patient, you should begin by examining them for low mood, starting with a general open enquiry and following up with more focused questions spanning the domains of biological, cognitive and behavioural symptomatology, including suicidality.

The good candidate will quickly observe that the symptomatology is, objectively speaking, rather sparse. In such circumstances it is important to satisfy yourself that the associated distress and/or disability is also minimal or absent.

If this is the case, you should then scrutinise the patient's health-seeking behaviour and determine whether it is understandable or 'normal' in terms of known personality and situational factors. If it is

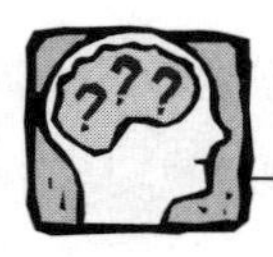

not, some other explanation must be sought (eg underlying psychosis, malingering, etc).

Explanation of findings

Once you have elicited the necessary information, deducing that the patient is not unwell is relatively straightforward. However, communicating this view may be more problematic. Given that the patient is a self-confessed worrier, it is important to offer reassurance that she is not suffering from a mental illness, and that her mild symptoms should resolve naturally with time. Avoid being dismissive of her difficulties – you should empathise with her predicament.

With regards to 'Prozac' you should advise that antidepressants are most effective when described for clinical depression of moderate or severe intensity. This patient does not have features of clinical depression, therefore is less likely to benefit from 'Prozac'. However, she would be at risk from adverse effects such as epigastric discomfort or sexual dysfunction.

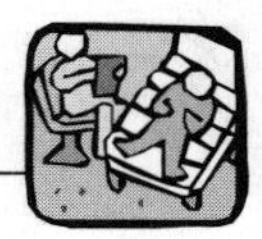

OSCE 42

Instructions for candidate

You have been asked to see the mother of a 22-year-old woman with an established diagnosis of bipolar affective disorder who is presenting with a manic episode. Please make an informant-based risk assessment. You have the permission of the patient. Explain your findings to the examiner.

Instructions for actor

You are the mother of a 22-year-old woman who has been diagnosed with bipolar affective disorder. Since she became unwell at the age of 19 years, your daughter has been admitted to hospital for psychiatric treatment on three occasions. The first admission was voluntary, after the patient herself sought help from the family GP, and was characterised by depressive symptoms associated with suicidal ideas of taking an overdose of tablets. During this admission you found a 'store' of over 100 paracetamol tablets apparently hidden in the patient's room at home. You assume that these were intended for use as an overdose, since as far as you are aware your daughter does not normally use this medicine. However, you have not felt able to confront her with this suspicion.

The last two admissions have been involuntary – that is, against the patient's will under the Mental Health Act – and have been characterised by classic manic symptoms, namely elated mood, grandiosity and overactivity. At these times your daughter has as you see it 'had quite a party', running up large debts on her credit card, using illicit substances, and having casual sex with strangers. On one such occasion she got into a fight with a bouncer outside a nightclub and sustained a black eye in the process. This kind of flamboyant and irresponsible behaviour is quite out of character for her.

Typically your daughter stops taking her medication in the period leading up to a manic episode, which on this occasion coincided with a new relationship, and during the episode itself, once established, she refuses to recommence treatment, insisting that she has 'never felt better'.

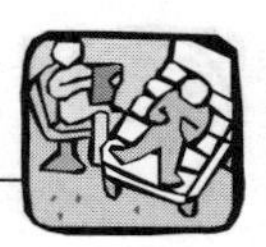

Construct

This OSCE is designed to test the candidate's ability to formulate a risk assessment in terms of seriousness, probability and associated risk factors, and to assign clinical priority accordingly. To achieve this, the candidate must exercise sufficient clinical skill to elicit the necessary information in a sensitive fashion.

Examiner's marking sheet

	Excellent	Good	Satisfactory	Fail	Poor
Communication skills and issues of confidentiality					
Identification of hazards and risk assessment					
Formulation of situational factors					
Overall mark					

Communication skills and issues of confidentiality

First you should explain the purpose of the interview, outlining what kind of information is being sought and why, and emphasising the need to keep the patient as safe from harm as possible.

Reassure the mother that you have the patient's informed consent and that any information which is provided will be treated confidentially and in the patient's best interests.

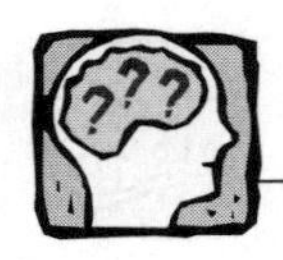

Identification of hazards and risk assessment

Begin with an open question addressing the mother's concerns about risks and harm. Take each risk identified in this way in turn, detailing and contextualising it as far as you can. Screen for any remaining risk behaviours, systematically covering the domains of risk to self from self, risk to others from self, and risk to self from others (vulnerability), and including acts of omission (eg self-neglect) as well as acts of commission (eg assault).

Formulation of situational factors

Based on the information available, the most serious risk would appear to be that of suicide. However, the immediate likelihood of this occurring would appear to be low, given that this risk is associated with depressive episodes.

The most pressing dangers concern the harms that accrue financially, socially and physically in association with the patient's manic relapses, which may be precipitated by non-compliance. Although taken individually these risks appear to be relatively minor, collectively and cumulatively they have the potential to lead to substantial disability unless they are checked. Moreover, the losses associated with the patient's manic episodes may herald a depressive downswing accompanied by the risk of suicide.

Further reading

Dolan, M & Doyle, M (2000). Violence risk prediction. Clinical and acturial measures and the role of the psychopathy checklist *British Journal of Psychiatry*, 177, 303–311.

Navneet Kapur (2000) Evaluating risks. *Advance Psychiatry Treatment*, November 2000, 6:399–406.

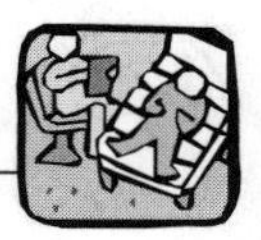

OSCE 43

Instructions for candidate

A GP has referred a 35-year-old employed man who is complaining of anxiety. Take a history of this man's presenting complaint. Explain your findings to the patient, including the most likely diagnosis. What further investigations would you wish to undertake?

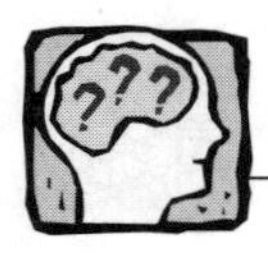

Instructions for actor

You are a happily married 35-year-old man who has recently been promoted to the position of assistant manager at the computing firm where you work.

Over the last three weeks you have been experiencing sudden unexpected and apparently unprovoked bouts of shortness of breath that last for about 5–10 minutes, associated with sweating, nausea, shaking, palpitations and the feeling that you are going to die. Understandably you are very concerned.

On consultation your GP has assured you that you are not in any mortal danger, but you are not convinced about this. If asked, you can confirm the absence of symptoms of diarrhoea, dizziness, weakness, headache or other pains, or pins and needles.

You are finding it difficult to adjust to your new occupational responsibilities. In particular, you dislike having to manage the performance of other people. If directly asked, you would admit to having always been a worrier who disliked change and felt awkward in new social situations, preferring his own company or that of close friends and family.

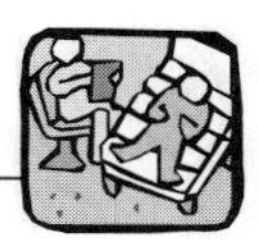

Construct

This OSCE is designed as a focused test of the candidate's knowledge of the symptomatology and aetiology of the anxiety and stress-related disorders, as well as their skills in communicating with an anxious patient.

Examiner's marking sheet

	Excellent	Good	Satisfactory	Fail	Poor
Communication skills					
Assessment of symptomatology					
Exploration of aetiology					
Explanation of investigations					
Overall mark					

Communication skills

When you have established rapport with the patient, you should follow up with an open question about the presenting complaint. You should then demonstrate to the examiners that you can apply a systematic and focused approach to the rest of your enquiry.

Assessment of symptomatology

For example, continue by screening for any remaining symptoms of anxiety, and then define the course and progression, identify any aetiological factors, and determine whether anything, including attempted treatments, has modified the illness for better or worse.

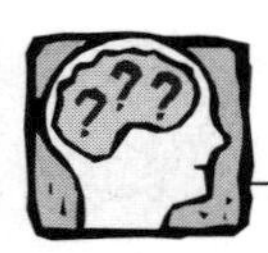

Explanation of aetiology and investigations

This process should lead you to the most likely formulation of a panic disorder precipitated by stress at work and predisposed by anxious/anankastic personality traits. However, it is important to bear in mind that there are other possibilities, including a mood disorder, a psychotic disorder, substance use or a physical condition.

You should be aware of this when communicating with the patient – in other words, emphasise that your diagnosis is provisional. However, given that the patient is by his own admission a worrier, it might be helpful even at this stage to offer a cognitive explanation for the genesis of his symptoms, namely somatic symptoms leading to fearful cognitions (eg 'I'm going to die'), thereby aggravating somatic symptoms, and so on.

Further investigations would include a full psychiatric history and examination, a physical examination, blood tests (including thyroid function), urinalysis (including drug screening) and an informant account.

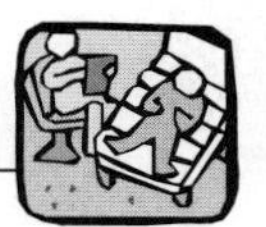

OSCE 44

Instructions for candidate

A 21-year-old woman with a suspected eating disorder has been referred by her GP. Calculate her body mass index (BMI) from the measurements and chart provided and make a brief assessment. Explain your findings to the patient. What further investigations would you like to perform?

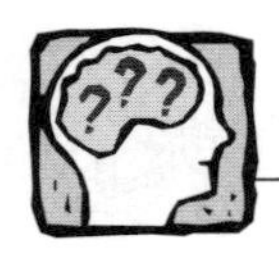

Instructions for actor

You are a 21-year-old woman who recently went to see your GP because of your concern about your weight and your increasingly desperate attempts to control it.

You recently started a new office job at a rather glamorous media organisation. You immediately began a rigorous diet but have struggled to maintain this. Over the last month you have been bingeing and vomiting every night and sometimes during the day as well.

If directly questioned you would admit to being a chubby child from a chubby family, but you had no concerns about your weight or shape until you reached 12 years of age, when you began dieting with friends 'for fun'. This activity gradually became more intense and frequent. However, although you find it is easy to lose weight, it is also easy to put it back on, which leaves you feeling bad about yourself. At such times you are seized by an irresistible urge to 'comfort eat', consuming up to five packets of chocolate biscuits on your own late into the night. After these 'binges' you typically feel bloated and disgusted with yourself, and this leads to secretive self-induced vomiting, after which you fall asleep. You regard yourself as 'overweight' but not 'fat'. However, you feel that if you could only 'be slim and stay slim', your life would be utterly transformed. Conversely, were you to become 'fat' you cannot imagine that life would be worth living. According to your bathroom scales you weigh 50 kg without your shoes. This is very close to your lowest ever recorded weight of 49 kg, and much better, you feel, than your peak weight of 60 kg. Your periods are regular.

Sometimes when you are alone and you think about your weight problems you feel miserable. However, such episodes rarely last longer than a few hours, when you are usually able to distract yourself by reading a magazine, watching a favourite television programme or phoning a friend. You enjoy your work, you think you are good at your job and popular, you have what you regard as an active social life, and you generally feel well and energetic. You only drink alcohol occasionally, and you never use illicit drugs, appetite suppressants or laxatives. You exercise twice a week at the local gym.

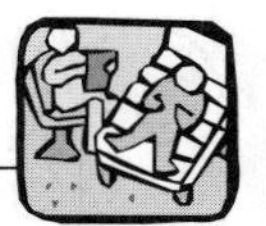

Equipment

- Weight and height centile chart
- Medical note recording a current height of 165 cm and a weight of 50.4 kg
- Calculator.

Construct

This OSCE assesses the candidate's general knowledge of eating disorders, and their ability to discriminate between different forms of eating disorder and to detect varying degrees of severity and comorbidity.

Examiner's marking sheet

	Excellent	Good	Satisfactory	Fail	Poor
Communication skills					
Eliciting core psychopathology					
Establishing the diagnosis					
Checking for comorbidity					
Correctly calculating body mass index					
Explanation of further investigation					
Overall mark					

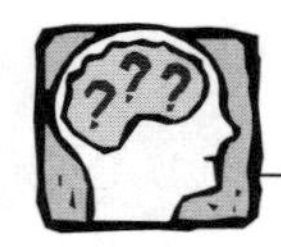

Communication skills

First of all, build a rapport with the patient, empathising with her. She will then be more willing to open up to you and talk with more confidence.

Core psychopathology and diagnosis

By their very nature, eating disorders lend themselves to objective measurement. Therefore they are likely to be encountered in OSCE examinations, and you should be prepared for them. Be aware of what BMI stands for (body mass index), its units (kg/m^2), how it is calculated (weight in kilograms divided by height squared in metres), the normal and threshold values, and how to measure height and weight correctly, should you be required to do so.

Fortunately, there is a limited number of defined syndromes, namely anorexia, bulimia and obesity with over-eating. Moreover, anorexia and bulimia share much core psychopathology (with which you should familiarise yourself), namely morbid over-valued ideation and distorted perceptions with regard to body size and shape. Likewise, you should ensure you have a thorough knowledge of the signs, symptoms and threshold values that distinguish these syndromes.

You need to know that a definite diagnosis of anorexia requires a substantial degree of weight loss (BMI < 17.5 or 15% below average for height) **and** the presence of associated endocrine complications (operationalised as amenorrhoea in women and impotence in men). In the absence of such signs, if there is a persistent morbid preoccupation with weight, and extreme measures are being taken in an attempt to lose weight (eg regular self-induced vomiting), combined with binge eating (episodes of craving followed by excessive uncontrolled consumption), a diagnosis of bulimia should be made. Remember that bulimia may occur in the presence of mild obesity.

Checking for comorbidity

Comorbidity tends to be the rule rather than the exception, complicating and sometimes clouding the diagnosis. You should screen for mood and personality factors and substance misuse. If such

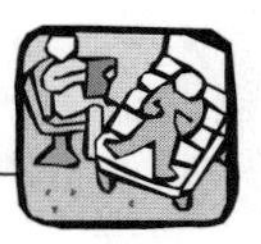

features are particularly prominent, you should consider whether in fact the eating pathology represents a subsidiary phenomenon. For example, there may be an underlying mood disorder. If your examination and in particular the history suggest that both an eating disorder and another disorder are present, you should list them separately and attempt to formulate the relationship between them.

Correctly calculating body mass index

In this OSCE the BMI is correctly calculated as 18.5 kg/m^2 – that is, above the threshold for anorexia, but below the ideal value. Likewise, there is an absence of amenorrhoea. However, the patient does appear to over-value thinness (her life would be 'utterly transformed' if she was 'thin'), and she has an exaggerated fear of being 'fat' (life would not be worth living). Moreover, her perception of her body size and shape would appear to be distorted in as much as she regards herself as overweight when in fact she is underweight. These features, taken together with the history of regular self-induced vomiting, are strongly indicative of a diagnosis of bulimia. For this patient, significant comorbidity can be excluded.

Exploration of further investigation

In any case of eating disorder it is important to consider non-psychological causes as well as complications from the disorder.

A full physical examination and blood tests, including a full blood count, urea and electrolytes, liver function, calcium and thyroid function are mandatory, especially if the weight changes are severe and the psychopathology is weak or poorly associated.

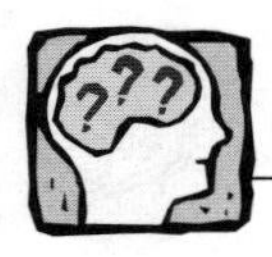

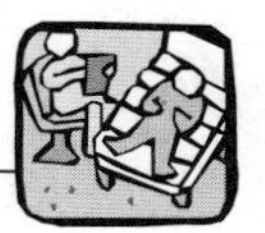

OSCE 45

Instructions for candidate

A 42-year-old man with a history of recurrent depression attends the outpatient clinic for a routine review. He appears to be well and tolerating a maintenance dose of antidepressant. Take a history of this man's personality. Explain your findings to the patient, including their significance (if any) for his mental illness. Are there any further investigations you would wish to undertake?

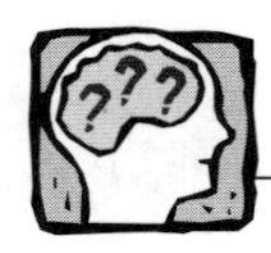

Instructions for actor

You are a 42-year-old accountant with a partner and two teenage children. For many years you have suffered from episodic severe depression, which on three occasions has been treated successfully with electroconvulsive therapy (ECT). Happily, you have remained well for the last four years on maintenance therapy with an antidepressant, without any adverse effects. Your last episode of illness coincided with a change of job following redundancy.

You would describe yourself as a quiet, thoughtful person who prefers the company of family and close friends. You like order and routine in both work and family life. For example, you insist that your partner and children use the bathroom at certain times only, according to a rota, and that when they do so they toilet, wash and groom themselves in a particular order. You become very upset if, for example, you go to use the bathroom during your allotted time slot only to find that it is occupied by your teenage daughter. Your daughter complains that she can never bring friends home because she finds all your household rules and regulations 'embarrassing'. More and more often your children appear to be flouting your rules, and this is leading to increasing family conflict.

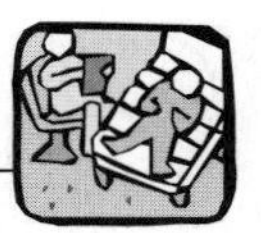

Construct

This OSCE assesses the candidate's knowledge of personality disorders and comorbidity in general, and the anankastic or obsessional subtype and depression in particular. It also tests the candidate's skill in efficiently screening for, detecting and defining personality disorders.

Examiner's marking sheet

	Excellent	Good	Satisfactory	Fail	Poor
Communication skills					
Comprehensively screening for personality subtypes					
Eliciting symptomatology					
Establishing subtype as a disorder					
Defining relationship with depression					
Overall mark					

Communication skills

Some preliminary explanation of why you are interested in assessing personality is probably in order here. You could say that in general in psychiatry it is important to know a person's personality so as to be able to judge whether there has been any change in habitual behaviour or attitude that might indicate that there is a mental health problem. More specifically, it is important to consider whether any pre-existing features of this patient's personality may be a factor in his illness or its treatment. Your task is not to make judgements about whether the patient is a good or a bad person, deserving or otherwise.

Screening for personality subtypes

Begin with an open question inviting the patient to describe himself 'as a person', that is his or her 'usual way of behaving, thinking and feeling, particularly towards others'. This may suggest the relevant sub-type or cluster of personality traits. In this case your initial inquiry should suggest anankastic/obsessive-compulsive traits belonging to the DSM IV Cluster C. However, before narrowing your focus it is important to screen for other personality trait groups or clusters, namely, Clusters A and B. A minimum of four conventional probes should be used including questions about the patient's sociability, mood/temper, coping style, and leisure interests. Research by Moran et al (2003) suggests it is helpful to probe as follows:

- Difficulty making and keeping friends
- Usually a loner
- Trusting others
- Normally loses temper easily
- Normally impulsive
- Normally a worrier
- Depends on others a lot
- Generally a perfectionist

Identifying the specific sub-type, eliciting symptomatology and establishing subtype for disorder

If a particular sub-type is suggested then the diagnosis should be pursued further with a comprehensive trait inquiry for that sub-type. In this case, screening should be followed up with more extended questions about obsessive traits including:

- feelings of excessive doubt; preoccupation with rules; perfectionism
- excessive conscientiousness; excessive adherence to social rules
- rigidity and stubbornness

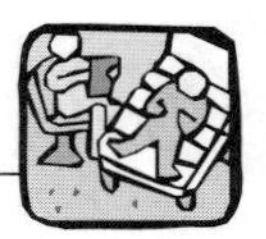

- unreasonable insistence that others conform to subject's way of doing things
- intrusion of insistent or unwelcome thoughts and impulses.

The presence of three or more such traits are diagnostic for the trait syndrome, however, the diagnosis of the disorder also requires that the traits are distressing or problematic in some way across a broad range of social and personal situations – this needs to be explicitly addressed with the patient.

Relationship to depression

The patient should be asked about whether he feels any aspect of his personality makes him vulnerable to depression, or whether he can see any pattern to his recurrent depressive episodes. Given the patient's personality profile you should have a high index of suspicion that his capacity to cope with change is poor, and, that therefore he would be particularly vulnerable to relapse around the time of significant life events, such as changing job or his children growing up and entering adolescence. If the patient does not volunteer this information himself it should be systematically sought. Conversely, in terms of the relationship between the patient's personality and his treatment it might be expected that this would be a beneficial one at least in so far as he is likely to be compliant with the treatment regimen – albeit obsessively so. Again, this should be explored in the interview.

Explanation to patient

You should explain to the patient that the indications are that he has a particular type of personality sometimes referred to as 'perfectionist' or 'obsessional'. You can reassure the patient that there is nothing 'wrong' with having this kind of personality; indeed there may be great benefits including conscientious and responsible attitudes to work and social life. However, such people tend not to tolerate change well, and this can lead to problems for them, for example, there is a known association with depressive illness. It may be that he is finding it difficult to cope with the increasing independence and assertiveness of his daughter's behaviour consequent upon them growing up. This may make him more vulnerable to relapse at this time.

Further investigation

A definitive diagnosis of personality disorder should never be made without the corroboration of a good informant, that is, someone who has known the patient well for at least five years, who is able and willing to give an accurate account. In this case the most obvious person to approach would be the patient's partner. Of course you would need to discuss this first with the patient and obtain his permission to proceed.

Further reading

Paul Moran, Morven Leese, Tennyson Lee, Paul Walters, Graham Thornicroft, Anthony Mann. **Standardised Assessment of Personality – Abbreviated Scale (SAPAS): preliminary validation of a brief screen for personality disorder.** *British Journal of Psychiatry*, September 2003; 183: 228 - 232.

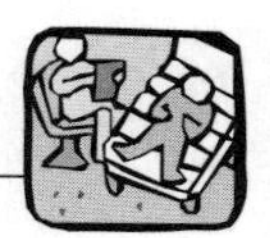

OSCE 46

Instructions for candidate

You are on a ward interviewing a patient with chronic schizophrenia. The patient was first diagnosed with schizophrenia several years ago and has been admitted on several occasions. His positive symptoms are controlled with anti-psychotic medication.

Take a history to illustrate the presence of the negative symptoms of schizophrenia.

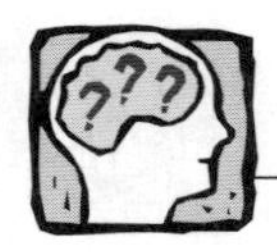

Instructions for actor

You are a 37-year-old man with schizophrenia. You are an inpatient on a psychiatric ward, receiving treatment for the voices that you hear. The medication seems to be working and you are looking forward to being discharged home. Concerns have been raised about your ability to look after yourself.

You are at risk of neglecting yourself. On the ward you need prompting to get out of your bed in the morning. Without further prompting, you would not wash yourself or tidy your room.

You need constant encouragement from the nursing staff in order for you to achieve anything constructive. You find it difficult to complete even simple tasks.

Most days you tend to sit alone in the smoking room for hours at a time. You don't like to engage in ward activities, despite the encouragement of the occupational therapist. Even when your family visits, you just sit in your chair and hardly say a thing.

You are co-operative with the doctor and you answer the questions briefly. Most of your answers are only one or two words long and you may also exhibit periods of silence. You sit impassively, with little spontaneous movement. Your face lacks emotional expression, your eye contact is poor and you look disinterested.

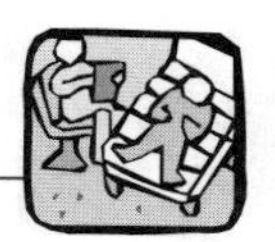

Construct

This station assesses the candidate's ability to elicit and identify the negative symptoms of schizophrenia.

Examiner's marking sheet

	Excellent	Good	Satisfactory	Fail	Poor
Communication skills					
Blunted emotions					
Lack of drive					
Relationship difficulties					
Overall mark					

Communication skills

The importance of using open questions initially and allowing the patient time to respond is shown in this scenario. A patient with chronic schizophrenia may exhibit a range of abnormalities in his communication abilities. He may be mute or show poverty of speech. The answers he gives may be vague and generalised. Periods of silence may also occur, either before answering a question or during a reply. Avoid interrupting or prompting the patient prematurely, otherwise you will miss these signs.

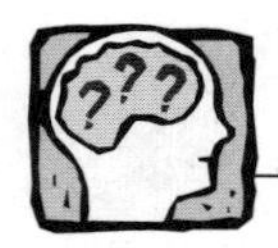

Blunted emotions

Many negative symptoms are expressed in the body language of patient and you may highlight these for the benefit of the examiner. The patient may sit still with little in the way of spontaneous movement. He may gaze blankly in no particular direction. Facial expressions may be limited and the patient's affect may not adjust to reflect his inner feelings. Eye contact may be reduced. The voice may be monotone or lack normal inflections.

Loss of drive

The patient may show a lack of motivation or goal-directed behaviour. Physical activity is limited and there is a reduced ability to experience pleasure. An interest in everyday activities such as personal grooming and cooking may be missing and there may be difficulties following an activity programme.

Relationship difficulties

Interpersonal relationships seem to be of little interest, so friendships become few and far between and the patient becomes increasingly isolated. Intimacy is reduced and sexual interest declines. Any relationships that do exist tend to be brief and superficial.

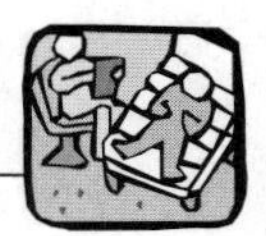

OSCE 47

Instructions for candidate

You are in the outpatient clinic talking to a lady with a history of panic attacks. She has asked you about how she can help herself because she is reluctant to take medication.

Explain relaxation techniques to this lady.

Instructions for actor

You are a 29-year-old woman with anxiety problems. A few times each week you become very anxious. You feel light-headed, your heart beats faster and harder, and you sweat a lot. You breathe faster and your chest feels tight. Sometimes your fingers tingle with 'pins and needles'.

The panic attacks happen at any time and at any place. Usually they last for a few minutes but they are very disabling. Consequently you are reluctant to go into public places for fear of embarrassing yourself.

You have decided to seek help by going to your family doctor who has sent you to see a psychiatrist because of the severity of your symptoms.

You appear both physically and mentally fine. You want to learn from the doctor how you can help yourself. You have heard about relaxation techniques and you want to learn more.

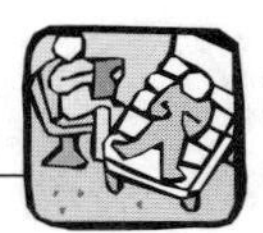

Construct

This station assesses the candidate's ability to explain relaxation techniques in a language that a lay person understands.

Examiner's marking sheet

	Excellent	Good	Satisfactory	Fail	Poor
Communication skills					
Progressive muscle relaxation					
Controlled breathing					
Guided imagery					
Offers supporting literature, relaxation tapes, or referral to an anxiety management group					
Overall mark					

Communication skills

Relaxation techniques are a useful skill for patients with mild to moderate anxiety symptoms to learn. When describing these techniques, give clear step-by-step instructions to the patient and check her understanding frequently. Asking the patient to repeat what you have just told her can be a useful indicator of how good your explanation was. Even better, you may demonstrate the techniques as you describe them and ask the patient to mirror your actions. There are a number of useful techniques and you should mention at least two you are familiar with.

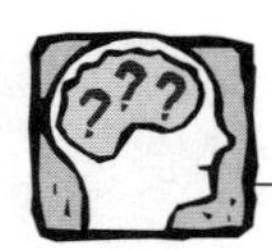

Progressive muscle relaxation

- Loosen your clothing and sit comfortably.
- Progressively work with groups of muscles. Start with the muscles in your hands, then move through your arms, shoulders, feet, legs, abdomen, back, neck and face.
- With each group of muscles, first tense the muscles, hold the tension for 10 seconds, and then relax them fully. Breathe in when you tense and breathe out when you relax. Pay attention to the difference in feeling between tension and relaxation.

Controlled breathing

- Sit comfortably, with your hands on your laps.
- Concentrate on your breathing, feel how the air flows in through your mouth, inflates the lungs and then flows back out.
- Breathe more slowly and more calmly. Concentrate on the movement of your chest wall as the air flows in and out.
- After each breath in, hold the breath for a few seconds before exhaling slowly.
- After a slow exhalation, leave your breath out for a few additional seconds. Let your muscles relax and allow the tension to slip away.

Guided imagery

- Sit comfortably, eyes closed.
  The goal is to visualise yourself in a peaceful environment, eg an exotic beach.
- 'Look' around the scene, adding details to the surroundings.
- Involve all five senses. For example, imagine the heat of the sun on your skin, the sounds of crashing waves, the coolness of the water, the smell of flowers.
- The more you practise, the more quickly you can imagine the complete scene and the quicker you will relax.

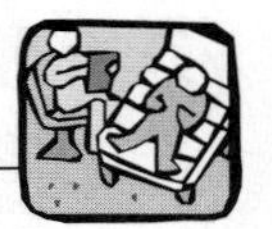

OSCE 48

Instructions for candidate

You are in casualty assessing a 19-year-old man. He is accompanied by his mother. He tells you that he has been having strange experiences in recent weeks. There have been at least five episodes in the last month and today he had another episode during which he was more disturbed. His mother witnessed today's episode and comments that he appeared 'vacant'.

Take a history of temporal lobe epilepsy from the patient.

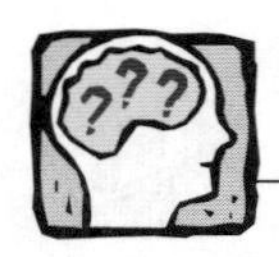

Instructions for actor

You are a 19-year-old man, living at home with your parents. Although you feel physically well, there have been some strange episodes in recent weeks.

During a typical episode, you have a funny feeling in your stomach and you feel sick. You start sweating and when you look in the mirror your face is red. When you look around the room, the surroundings appear unreal. You feel detached from yourself. Your heart beats harder and faster and you feel scared and emotional. Within a few minutes, the episode ends.

On one occasion you remember seeing the furniture around you but the objects were distorted in size and shape. On two occasions, you had a strange taste in your mouth even though you were not eating anything at the time and there was a foul odour in the room. You don't know how to explain this.

Today you had another episode. You were in the company of your mother. She told you that you were staring into space and appeared vacant, not responding to her call. You were smacking your lips and swallowing. You cannot recall this yourself but you remember feeling confused after the episode and your mother standing over you shouting your name. It was as if you had been daydreaming for a few minutes.

You have never bitten your tongue or suffered with incontinence during an episode. You have never been diagnosed with epilepsy.

You co-operate with the doctor and answer the questions appropriately. You comment to the doctor that you have a sense of déjà vu – ie a sense of familiarity with the casualty department even though you have never been here before. You are concerned that you are going mad.

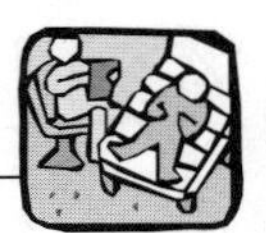

Construct:

This station assesses the candidate's ability to break bad news to a carer.

Examiner's marking sheet

	Excellent	Good	Satisfactory	Fail	Poor
Communication skills					
Takes a history of auras					
Takes a history of, and differentiates between, simple and complex partial seizures					
Excludes other psychiatric and behavioural disorders					
Overall mark					

Communication skills

You need to be very tactful when breaking news to the carer.

Aura and seizures

- Simple or complex partial seizures occur in temporal lobe epilepsy, not grand mal seizures.
- During a simple partial seizure, consciousness is preserved but the patient may experience an aura which is a range of symptoms, including:

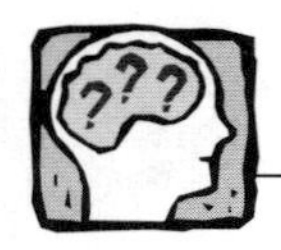

- Autonomic symptoms, such as nausea, sweating, flushing of the face, an increase in the heart rate, piloerection and epigastric sensations, often reported as 'stomach rising' or a 'funny feeling in my stomach'.
- Intense sudden emotion not related to events at the time.
- Hallucinations and/or illusions, in any sensory modality, including objects appearing distorted in size, shape and distance.
- Sensations of déjà vu, jamais vu, derealisation and depersonalisation.

The complex partial seizure typically has a relatively gradual indistinct onset, developing over a couple of minutes and lasting up to 10 minutes. Consciousness is impaired in complex partial seizures. The patient tends to have a motionless stare (the absence) accompanied by automatisms, which are stereotyped, repetitive, involuntary movements, such as oro-alimentary (lip smacking, chewing or swallowing without a cause) or gestural (fumbling, fidgeting, picking up objects, abnormal movements of the head, scratching, walking, running). Vocalisation is also common. There may be loss of memory about the events around a complex partial seizure and a period of post-ictal confusion, which distinguishes temporal lobe epilepsy from absence seizures.

Excludes other psychiatric and behavioural disorders

Because of the overlap of symptoms with other psychiatric disorders, such as affective and psychotic illnesses, you should ask screening questions to confirm the diagnosis of temporal lobe epilepsy and exclude the differential diagnoses.

Index

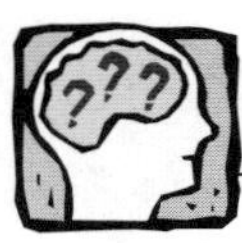

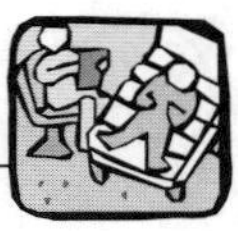

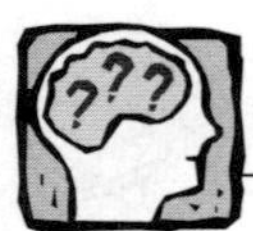

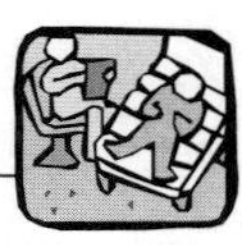

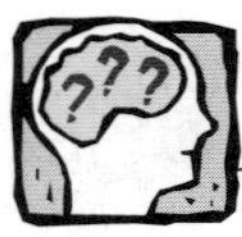

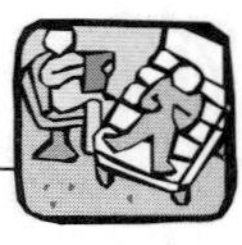

T

V

W

Z